T MYTHOLOGY N LAW

The Mythology of Modern Law is a radical reappraisal of the role of myth in modern society. Peter Fitzpatrick uses the example of law, as an integral category of modern social thought, to establish the relevance and centrality of myth in modernity.

Peter Fitzpatrick argues that law is mythic, both in its origin and as a continuing social force, and that it depends for its identity on other mythic categories, such as the nation, the individual and 'the sciences of man and society'. He traces the development of the hold of mythology on Western society back to the Enlightenment, despite the supposedly secular rationality of that period, and shows how it was strengthened by the experience of imperialism, when European identity was created in opposition to racially defined 'others'.

Challenging and controversial, *The Mythology of Modern Law* questions current conceptions of legal and social theory. It revises the very foundations of jurisprudence and the sociology of law and undermines the exclusive stands taken within these disciplines. An invaluable reference for all debates surrounding modernity, post-modernity and law, the book will also be of great interest to those concerned with the history of European racism.

Peter Fitzpatrick is Professor of Law and Social Theory at the University of Kent.

SOCIOLOGY OF LAW AND CRIME
Editors:
Maureen Cain, *University of the West Indies*
Carol Smart, *University of Leeds*

This new series presents the latest critical and international scholarship in sociology, legal theory, and criminology. Books in the series will integrate the sociology of law and the sociology of crime, extending beyond both disciplines to analyse the distribution of power. Realist, critical, and postmodern approaches will be central to the series, while the major substantive themes will be gender, class and race as they affect and, in turn, are shaped by legal relations. Throughout, the series will present fresh theoretical interpretations based on the latest empirical research. Books for early publication in the series deal with such controversial issues as child custody, criminal and penal policy, and alternative legal theory.

THE MYTHOLOGY
OF MODERN LAW

Peter Fitzpatrick

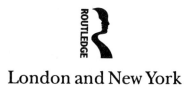

London and New York

First published in 1992
by Routledge
11 New Fetter Lane, London EC4P 4EE

Simultaneously published in the USA and Canada
by Routledge
a division of Routledge, Chapman and Hall Inc.
29 West 35th Street, New York, NY 10001

Typeset by LaserScript, Mitcham, Surrey
Printed and bound in Great Britain
by Biddles Ltd, Guildford and King's Lynn

British Library Cataloguing in Publication Data
A catalogue record for this book is available from the British Library.

Library of Congress Cataloging in Publication Data
Fitzpatrick, Peter, 1941–
The mythology of modern law/Peter Fitzpatrick.
p. cm. – (Sociology of law and crime)
Includes bibliographical references (p.   ) and index.
1. Sociological jurisprudence. 2. Myth. I. Title. II. Series.
K370.F57 1992
340'.115 – dc20   92-296
CIP

ISBN 0–415–04380–8
0–415–08263–3 (pbk)

For Anne O'Donovan

CONTENTS

PREFACE

Modernity, for a start, is not supposed to be about myth. Nor can a sober and secular law any longer inhabit the realm of the sacred. The very idea of myth typifies 'them' – the savages and ancestors 'we' have left behind. Myth now can only be a residue or an aberration, a faint evocation of paradise lost or a resurgence of monsters. In the infinite arrogance of modernity, myth is made to correspond with the static and closed in meaning and social ordering whilst modernity is equated with progress and a fecund openness. Yet the origins and identity of modern society are still described in seemingly mythic terms, in terms of the division between us and them, culture and nature, and so on. But these terms can no longer be mythic. They can no longer represent fixed limits for they are now caught up in a progression of the boundless project of modernity where limits can only be temporary restraints pending further discovery or more effective manipulation. Modernity, in short, is opposed to myth.

In my argument, that stand is inverted. No matter what its relevance to so-called primitive and ancient worlds, myth is vibrantly operative in modernity. It is not confined to the fitful traces of antiquity nor is it a matter of mythopoeic aspiration. The obvious conundrum, then, is how this presence of myth can be reconciled with its denial in modernity. The answer is that the denial is the myth. The mythology of European identity is founded in an opposition to certain myth-ridden 'others'. These are constructed not as the exemplary affirmations of a classic mythology but in terms of a negative teleology: 'so far as I know, we are the only people who think themselves risen from savages: everyone else believes they descend from Gods' (Sahlins 1976: 52–3). Occidental being is impelled in a progression away from aberrant

ix

origins. It is formed in the comprehensive denial of the 'other' – in assertions of universal knowledge, imperious judgement and encompassing being. Since it is constructed in negation, in terms of what it is not, this being is unbounded and able mythically to reconcile its particular and contingent existence with its appropriation of the universal.

The mythology of modernity is sustained in the experience of imperialism. Nowadays, imperialism is usually seen as something marginal, exceptional and evanescent, whereas in my argument it is central, ordinary and enduring. True, there is a certain amnesic quality associated with imperialism and the mythology it engenders. But, to extend Nietzsche's conception somewhat, 'oblivion is not merely a *vis inertiae*, as is often claimed, but an active screening device'; this 'active oblivion' is a constructive forgetting which serves to constitute what is remembered, what is real and effective (Nietzsche 1956: 189 – Second Essay – Part I). There results, in Derrida's precisely ambiguous term, a 'white mythology' – the mythology of a whitened Europe and a mythology leached somewhat of its original, fabulous colour (Derrida 1982: 213). Such a process does not mark the decline of myth but rather its perfection, its more extensive entry into social and self organization. The Occident becomes imbued with that very totality of commitment to myth and with that unresponsiveness to a wider world which it so readily and wrongly attributes to the primitives and the ancients.

Modern law is a form of this white mythology. It shares origins and a sustaining dynamic with the general mythology of modernity and it is a key character in that mythology. The mythic composition of law can be made out in its contradictory attributes. Law is autonomous yet socially contingent. It is identified with stability and order yet it changes and is historically responsive. Law is a sovereign imperative yet the expression of a popular spirit. Its quasi-religious transcendence stands in opposition to its mundane temporality. It incorporates the ideal yet it is a mode of present existence. In a time of unabashed myth, these persistent irresolutions, the very stock-in-trade of jurisprudential debate, could be readily reconciled in various yet related realities. But this resolution is not explicitly available in a modernity where reality is unified and truth indivisible. What is more, law typifies a modern form of rational authority that rejects the division of life between different mythic realms (see Kronman 1983: 47). In short, the enduring contradictions about law correspond to its mythic dimensions, yet these cannot be recognized in a non-mythic world. I aim to accord them recognition and to show how such contradictions cohere in myth.

Mythologies have to be set and the scene I am describing is variously British and English with their imperial extensions. But I am not concerned with 'the peculiarities of the English' and the particular mythology of the law emerging from the Germanic forests, Saxon moots and various other locations (cf. Pocock 1967). My concern is with the British scene as a case or an instance of an Occidental mythology shared with much of continental Europe and North America. I have, therefore, ranged more widely than Britain in constructing my counter-myth.

Peter Fitzpatrick
Canterbury
Autumn 1991

SERIES EDITORS' PREFACE

This series owes a great deal to Peter Fitzpatrick's *The Mythology of Modern Law*. This happy debt is both historical and contemporary.

In the tangled and complex negotiations with various publishers which led to the establishment of the series Peter participated as an adviser and at one time a likely co-editor. His plan for the *Mythology* constituted a major selling point of our proposal to launch a fully integrated series, in which feminist work and scholarship compatible with feminist thinking would appear together. So, we argued, the ghettoization of feminist work could be ended if not transcended. The *Mythology* more than adequately fills this intellectual and political bill. It is not 'on, by, or for' women. But the analysis it develops to demonstrate the integral and foundational character of racism in law reveals a space and an opportunity for a sister analysis of women's continuously marginal standing as full legal 'persons'.

Like the authors whom Peter Fitzpatrick berates, we have begun this Preface to *Mythology* by saying what it is not. Happily, however, we are also in a position to say what it is, and herein lies our current indebtedness.

First, this is a book which de-constructs the Occidental myths which found and permeate law. Myth is a form which unifies without (apparently) totalizing, a form which maintains unity in apparent inconsistency, and presence in apparent absence. This is a book, then, which reveals that mythology is not extant only in 'other' societies, but pervasive in our own, and perhaps most potent in those places where its absence is most loudly proclaimed, that is to say in those twin sites of reason and hard headedness, the law and the sciences.

Second, this is a book which explains the racism of neutral and

SERIES EDITORS' PREFACE

racially indifferent legality. We have wrestled in our own work with
the problem of how equal justice – and sometimes it *is* even-
handedly dispensed – leads to profoundly unequal outcomes, with
more and longer prison sentences for black than for Caucasian
people in the UK, for example. Fitzpatrick reveals how law depends on racism for its own theory of its being, not only for its self
justification (though for that too) but for its very identity, which is
achieved in negation, by the distinction between a legal way of
doing coercion and all other ways. These out-lawed and un-lawed
ways mark and constitute these others as savages or despots. And
yet their lawlessness is deemed to precede the Law, which
'developed' from these unpromising origins into what the origins
are not.

Racism, as Fitzpatrick demonstrates, is foundational, and as
much so in contemporary legal theory as it was in the Enlightenment.

In making clear the mode of operation of negative definitions
this book provides another invaluable base not just for understanding the law, the legal subject, civil or 'civilised' society, but
also any negatively defined phenomenon. The influence of
Durkheim and the French tradition that remains in Foucault
(repressive to restitutive law, for example), persists as a trace in
Fitzpatrick. Durkheim's definition of crime is a negative one,
capable of being exploited by officials and others to suit the
occasion. But in both Foucault and Fitzpatrick the functionalism
and optimism have gone, to be replaced by a hoped-for resistance
which becomes more and more difficult as the techniques for
normalizing 'wayward' identities become discursively and admini-
stratively more sophisticated day by day.

The work of negative definition does not stop there, however.
Fitzpatrick explores the consequences of the infinite possibilities
which negative definition allows. Thus, in relation to administration (or regulatory law), the effective policing of both its boundaries and its content is achieved by 'law' while that same law
acknowledges a terrain of expertise and science which it does not
authorize itself to tamper with. This is the zone of the self-
legitimating knowledge of the non-accountable expert, brought
into being by and deploying the technical discourses of positive
power. Fitzpatrick's point is that the negative definition of law
allows law to be limited by administration without losing legal face
and too while retaining the situationally flexible power to decide

xiii

who is an expert and what the acceptable boundaries of that expertise may be at any time.

Not only does this connect with the formal versus substantive justice debate which has enlivened and bedevilled both juris-prudence and sociology since Weber, not only does it resolve the dilemma of politically consequential slippage between categories for informal justice theorists, it also secures all the categories in Foucault's more general theory of (or discourse about) social order itself. This is achieved by using the Foucauldian concept of administration to characterize the wide range of forms of in-corporated and regulatory justice that have been identified and discussed with increasing fervour throughout this century.

We have said nothing yet about Progression, that most open-ended of objectives, that most amenable justification, when read backwards, for all past practices. We have said nothing about nationhood, also foundationally conceived in difference, or the disorder creating properties of law in the colonial setting and the working class home. We have said nothing about the concealed coercions of popular justice. We have even – and this must be a record – we have even said nothing about H.L.A. Hart, who warrants a chapter of his own to demonstrate that the foundational mythologies are alive and well and living in the twentieth century.

But it is not the task of an editorial Preface either to summarize or to review the book. What we have done is to situate this major contribution within the discipline (sic) of sociology of law and within the series. We invite you now to read it, to enjoy it, and to be both angered by what it reveals, and stimulated by the intel-lectual and conceptual music it makes.

Maureen Cain
Carol Smart
January 1992

ACKNOWLEDGEMENTS

Much generosity and kindness went into the making of this book. It was first mapped out during an exciting semester spent in 1987 at the invitation of Carleton University with its Departments of Law and Sociology. It broadened in discussions with Hans Mohr which he made as expansive as that reach of the St Lawrence River where we talked. And it was given much initial impetus in Alan Hunt's magnanimous concern. With its more immediate production, there was the pleasure of working again with Maureen Cain. Elisabeth Tribe was the most supportive and effective of editors. Elleke Boehmer, Tony Carty, Dave Reason, Leon Schlamm, David Sugarman and Bernard Sharratt offered apt references at apt moments. Deborah Cheney and Rachael Reilly helped creatively with the research. Nancy Fulton and Peter Goodrich commented cogently on parts of the manuscript. Liz Cable put it all together to perfection and Tesher Fitzpatrick similarly organized the references. Colin Perrin provided the exemplary index and Valerie Mendes for Routledge was a committed copy-editor. To Shelby Fitzpatrick, I remain more grateful than it is possible to say.

I have drawn on and reworked two published pieces. Part of chapter 5 is derived from 'The Impossibility of Popular Justice' published in *Social and Legal Studies* (1992), and much of chapter 6 is a development of my contribution to *Dangerous Supplements* published by Pluto Press and Duke University Press (1991).

1

MYTH AND THE NEGATION
OF LAW

The primary aim of the critic is to see the object as it is really not.
(Wilde in Ellmann 1988: 137)

INTRODUCTION

The suspiciously simple argument of this chapter is that law as a
unified entity can only be reconciled with its contradictory existences if we see it as myth. Such a claim may appear at first to
compound contradiction. Modern law, after all, was formed in the
very denial of that mythic realm which had so deluded the pre-
moderns. My summary response is to agree but then to say that
such a denial typifies a renewed and now modern mythology. In
this negation of mythic being, there is a denial of that which gives
law coherent existence. Negation through law is the negation of
law. Yet, as I show in later chapters, it is this negative quality, this
vacuity of law, which enables a mythic mediation to be effected
between law's contradictory existences and which enables the
unity of law to be maintained.

Beginnings are always desperate. To sustain one already so
comprehensively set in negation could prove peculiarly awkward.
It may be better to start again. Borrowing a beginning from
Foucault borrowing from Borges, there is a 'certain Chinese encyclopaedia' which, in classifying animals, begins '(a) belonging to
the Emperor, (b) embalmed,' proceeds via '(e) sirens, (f) fabulous, (g) stray dogs', and ends '(m) having just broken the water
pitcher, (n) that from a long way off look like flies' (Foucault 1970:
xv). What Borges does here is to dispense 'with the least obvious,
but most compelling, of necessities; he does away with the *site*, the
mute ground upon which it is possible for entities' to co-exist as a

1

classification which 'we' can understand (Foucault 1970: xvii – his emphasis).

Another provocation to discover the mute ground can be derived from the treatment of diversity in scientific fields. Take the not uncommon scientific controversy where seemingly opposed positions each supported by 'unassailably "objective" evidence' are both shown to be 'valid': an example would be 'the complementarity principle of Bohr, affirming the right of coexistence of both a corpuscular and a wave concept of light' (Weiss in Merton 1981: iv). What may be the case, Merton believes, is that in 'each field of inquiry . . . the plurality of current theories, paradigms, and thought-style are not mere happenstance . . . . Rather, it appears to be integral to the socially patterned cognitive processes operating in the discipline' (Merton 1981: v). When these processes are made explicit, they can reveal a unity in a field which previously seemed to be made up of diverse accounts. To take an instance: differing accounts of human evolution in paleoanthropology can become congruent when they are all seen as versions of the one myth (Landau 1991). In more conventional terms, we may agree that scientific advance often results, as in particle physics, from positing then seeking to discover an entity which would unify diverse but co-existing entities in the field. Contrawise, the accepted unity of a field may depend on connections operating but unrecognized within it (cf. Sheldrake 1981).

Myth, I will argue, is the mute ground which enables 'us' to have a unified 'law' and which brings together law's contradictory existences into a patterned coherence. That coherence extends beyond Merton's 'cognitive processes' and beyond the psychological categories to which myth in the modern period is usually subordinated, when it is recognized at all – categories of belief or of unconscious projection. Rather, the myth pursued here is every bit as sociologically elaborated as that which supposedly bound the primitives and the ancients. I will begin to develop the argument by indicating an intriguing paradox about law. There would seem to be a consensus on the object 'law' extending over the otherwise divergent accounts of it (see Duxbury 1987: 29–31, 189–207; Sargent 1991). Some common conception appears to be compatible, for example, with both the sociology of law and the focus on legal doctrine. Yet the conflict between these two positions is supposedly fundamental. Jurisprudence is littered with isolated and opposed notions about law but the field retains a unity of engagement with law. To the extent that the keepers of one notion engage with another, it is to reduce that other notion to the terms of their own. Further thought and the accumulation of knowledge will eventually establish the rightness of one position over or rather than another. The immensity of effort so far unsuccessfully devoted to this consummation suggests that persistent irresolution is a more likely outcome. Might it not be that in such persistence there are enduring if opposed elements of law; and if we grant this, how can the opposition then be reconciled with a unified law? Obviously, I will be seeking the answer in myth. Obviously also, I cannot fairly accommodate all the mutually opposed conceptions of law. I will, instead, begin looking for an answer in an opposition that encompasses many others and marks the major divide in modern jurisprudence – that is, the opposition between law as autonomous doctrine and law as dependent on society.

THE ASSUMPTION OF LAW

Seeing law as autonomous doctrine is supposedly the antithesis of social approaches to law. The doctrinal study of law – or, in cognate terms, black-letter law, formalism or legal positivism – takes legal rules and reports of cases as the universe. This approach remains predominant in legal education and legal research. Ostensibly, it renders law as distinct, unified and internally coherent (Sugarman 1991: 34–5). In its guise of analytical or positivist jurisprudence, it has assiduously protected law's autonomy. Numerous, seemingly devastating assaults on this position have failed fundamentally to alter it. The remorseless observation of its divergence from the practice of law has not undermined the standard perception of its place at the foundation of that practice.

The form which this approach has recently taken within jurisprudence has been that of the elevation of the heroic champion – the champion as both protector of true knowledge and the predominant figure in the field. The champion's conceptual defence of law's autonomy is promulgated and refined but eventually found wanting in some ways. The new champion's rise is effected by the discovery of ways which significantly qualify the old position and by the provision of some generally acceptable protection of law's autonomy to put in its place. The current champion remains H. L. A. Hart with his 'concept of law' (Hart 1961). The leading challenger is Ronald Dworkin with his notion of 'law's empire'

(Dworkin 1986). I will briefly consider each of these as intimations of myth.

Hart attacked the long dominant, and still influential, positivist conception of law provided by John Austin. Austin saw law as the command of a sovereign power which is generally obeyed by the populace: the relation between the sovereign and members of society is one of simple dependence (Austin 1861–3: 1, 170–1 – I). By paying some regard to sociolinguistic usage, Hart finds Austin's conception to be deficient on several grounds. Most significantly, it ignores the various social uses of legal rules (Hart 1961: 88). If we regard these, we find that people have an 'internal', participating approach to law in which they adopt a creative, reflective attitude to legal rules. We find them endowed with abilities to act on and evaluate legal standards of behaviour and to pursue the highly skilled enterprise of rule-following (Hart 1961: 55–6, 96). This popular element proves, in Hart's analysis, to be essential for law's being. Having inserted this popular element into law so as to displace the current positivist champion, Hart proceeds to assume his mantle in a mystifying shift. Hart erases the element of the popular and reaffirms the positivist equation of law with official authority and with formal, pre-set meaning. The populace is thus excluded from law and relegated to a state of Austinian inertness. Hart achieves all this through forms of the mythic elevation of law and of the official voice as the source of law. The popular element is silenced in a fabulous story of law's primal origin. I will consider all this in more detail in chapter 6 on 'law as myth'. In short, what counts as law becomes exclusively and comprehensively determined by officials and the positivist enterprise is preserved.

Dworkin follows a path which parallels Hart's remarkably. He equates Hart's conception of law with a system of rules and then finds it inadequate because it does not accommodate other things integral to 'our own practices' in law (Dworkin 1968: 60). In particular, the idea of a rule cannot include the use of principles in judicial decision-making. Principles, however, import an unsettling social dimension into law, thereby challenging its autonomy. Principles, as Dworkin recognizes, have a more extensive existence than that reflected in law (see e.g. Dworkin 1968: 51). How then can law's reliance on principles be reconciled with its autonomy?

The great answer eventually found by Dworkin lay in interpretation. This does not, at first, appear to be an auspicious resolution. The recent revival of interpretation in several academic fields has revealed the contingent or dependent nature of things usually assumed to have an autonomous existence. Nor does Dworkin seem to stint in his adoption of interpretation. With his consolidating work on *Law's Empire*, Dworkin sees that empire as 'defined' simply by 'an interpretative, self-reflective attitude': 'Law is an interpretive concept, which does not have an identity apart from the activity of interpreting law' (Dworkin 1986: 410, 413). In ways Dworkin is true to such a promiscuous and decidedly non-imperial basis for law. Seeing law as interpretative activity leads him to adopt an 'internal, participants' point of view' on law (Dworkin 1986: 14). Participants comprise 'every actor in the practice' of law and all 'people who have law', such as 'citizens and politicians and law teachers' (Dworkin 1986: 13–14). To equate law with the diversity of participants' perspectives is a truly radical step, one which would spectacularly justify Dworkin's constant claim to be opposed to positivist jurisprudence. Yet this paradox-ically diffuse empire soon assumes a more conventionally imperial dimension. By the end of Dworkin's account, law has acquired a singular voice and a posited identity distinct from the diversity of interpretation. In the affirmation of empire, law becomes the preserve of officials who have 'the last word', even if the word is infused with the strivings of legal philosophers – the 'seers and prophets' of the law (Dworkin 1986: 407, 413). There is mystery as to how such a transformation takes place (Duncanson 1989; Hunt and Kerruish: in press). The answer lies in operative forces infus-ing law – forces of infinite competence, perfectibility and cohering order. These forces elevate a particular and official interpretation of law and invest this law with abilities and values which render it transcendent and constant. Law is thus accorded a singularity and inviolability which more than match the efforts of prior positivists to secure its autonomy. As with Hart – as with Austin – law exists because 'officials . . . take . . . decisions that commit a community to rights and duties that make up law' (Dworkin 1986: 97).

The relation between law's autonomy and society in these ac-counts is thus somewhat paradoxical. With both Hart and Dworkin, law's social being serves to reveal the inadequacy of the reigning positivist conception of law. That conception is shown to be inextricably dependent on a social dimension. But when it came to purifying law and sustaining the positivist enterprise, the social dimension was arbitrarily excluded and law's dependence proved to be readily, if mysteriously, extricable. Law could thence occupy a transcendent position where it has no specific connection with society but nonetheless exercises a general domination over it. Positivist domination has to be constantly secured in the face of social challenges that would render law as something apart from what it is posited to be. Both Hart and Dworkin adopt their particular, limiting participants' perspective partly to counter 'external' or 'pragmatic' perspectives that would reduce law in terms of social factuality (Dworkin 1986: 95; Hart 1961: 78).

The opposition that this imports between positivist and social accounts of law is very much overdrawn: the position of law in social accounts is not so simple and neither is it any less paradoxical than in positivist jurisprudence. The gist of these social accounts is usually taken to be that law, rather than dominating society, is itself wholly a product of society. It changes as society changes and it can even disappear when the social conditions that created it disappear or when they change into conditions antithetical to it. A pervasive administration and a renewed community are the social forms usually taken as effecting or resulting from the end of law (see e.g. Unger 1976). Yet if we observe these social accounts more closely, we can find a law that seems to be secure and persistent. The contradiction between this seeming autonomy and law's social dependence is resolved, I argue, in the mythic elevation of law. The relation between law and such social forms as administration and community can thence be seen as a relation between mutually supporting mythic entities and not simply as one of opposition. But this is to anticipate much of my later argument and to summarize its detailed illustration in chapter 5. For the moment, I will pursue law and its distinct identity in these social accounts.

With some of these accounts the pursuit is too easy and need not take long. These are accounts from within law – accounts which take law as given and see its relation to society in such instrumental terms as bringing about change, problem-solving and policy implementation, or simply in terms of effectiveness. Thus, 'socio-legal studies' is an area usually seen as conducive to 'understandings of the workings of law and to law's effectiveness': in this exercise 'sociologists should be on tap but not on top' (see Nelken 1981: 36). There are other influential approaches broadly of this type. Sociological jurisprudence, for example, is essentially a view from within law. It is concerned with law's effectiveness and with its capacity for 'social engineering', even if these concerns are, as it were, allowed to reflect back on the nature of law. This approach reaches something of an elaborated terminus in the work of Julius Stone (Stone 1966). The perspective called law in context provides a currently influential and more diverse instance. In some of its reaches, it is indistinguishable from conventional socio-legal studies, but it is sometimes concerned with the constitution of law in terms of context. Yet, as the name implies, law in context tends to posit a constant law in varying contexts.

Law's singular presence is only somewhat less conspicuous in approaches that would thoroughly constitute law in terms of society, or see it as essentially dependent on society, or require it to be in phase with society. The sociology of law, to take the most prominent approach, has a large respect for general sociology but it confronts law narrowly, leaving it intact and even reinforced in law's own terms. The mode of this confrontation is usually functionalist. Law is explained by the function it performs and in this it is seen as having a straightforward relation of effectiveness in its impact on behaviour, or in social change (see Black 1976). Functionalism simply assumes a constituting relationship between law and function. To indicate the limits of this approach, I will take the common attribution to law of the function of conflict resolution. Far from resolving conflict, law will often provide modes and occasions for its creation, expression and perpetuation, for sustaining one sphere of life in enduring conflict with another. Resolution may lie in the systematic nature of the conflict and in some other institutional site besides law, such as exchange (see e.g. Strathern 1985). Persistent conflict, rather than generating or invoking law, may sustain incompatibilities and indeterminancies that make legal resolution impossible. Anthropological accounts fare no better than the sociology of law. In concentrating doggedly on the functional category of dispute resolution, either the issue of constituting law is avoided altogether or we encounter the same difficulties as those just instanced for sociology. In the older tradition of comparative anthropology, the aim is certainly to fix law's universal social character but this is done, unwittingly or otherwise, by taking attributes of Western law as given and reading them back into a supposed evolutionary or historical record (see Fitzpatrick 1985).

There are other sociological and evolutionary denials of law's distinct identity and I will return to these in chapter 4. For the moment I will conclude this survey with the strongest and most intensely debated denial: that provided by Marxism. The terms of the debate have become rather worn but the outcome, or lack of it, remains instructive. A so-called vulgar and instrumental Marxism saw law as epiphenomenal. Its being was determined by an economic base or by its utility in class domination. That supposed position has never existed far from a concern with the autonomy of social forms (see e.g. Marx 1973: 102–6). The usual response to an impertinent autonomy was to locate it within the determining dynamic or structure. Thus, with Pashukanis, the seemingly autonomous form of law is a product of commodity exchange conceived of in a Marxist frame – but Pashukanis also recognized that this was not a comprehensive notion of law (Pashukanis 1978: chapter 4). In the once greatly influential variant provided by Althusser, law would have a quasi-autonomy created by its part within a determining structure (e.g. Althusser 1971: 124–49). This provided an origin for the once closely observed idea of law's relative autonomy but, with the undermining of the encompassing structure (see Hindess and Hirst 1977), nothing else was found to which the autonomy could be made relative. Law was left without any constraining connections to which it could be related. There followed a constant and still current advocacy on the 'left' of law's self-sustained existence. Law had to be 'taken seriously' or one had to be sturdily 'realistic' about its necessity. Thus a 'responsible socialism' – entailing much responsibility and little socialism – would exhort us to be realistic about the necessity for criminal law, and this not only because people are against crime and people have votes, but also because such law will in some ways have to be maintained in a future socialist society (see Cottrell 1984). This was a socialism of a broad or uncertain dispensation which could no longer be assuredly anticipated. In all, law no longer occupied a constraining structure or history.

Intellectually, the end of these various searchings for law's comprehensively defining social foundation is marked by the 'constitutive theory' of law developed mainly in critical legal studies. In his seminal contribution, Klare, after rehearsing dissatisfactions with Marxist reductions of law, proceeded to discover that law acts on, even constitutes, society (Klare 1979; see also Poulantzas 1978: 83, 87). Furthermore, law and society inextricably yet somehow distinctly constitute and inhabit each other (see e.g. Harrington and Yngvesson 1990). With the constitutive theory, there can no longer be any inexorable mode or structure of connecting law to society. There is an ascendant resolution of this division which brings matters full circle. Autopoiesis is a social account of law, yet one which would hermetically secure law by according it the self-creating power to absorb and order society in its own terms (see e.g. Teubner 1989). Quite apart from its particular virtues, auto-poiesis can sustain its seemingly extravagant claim for law because it incorporates what I now indicate is a myth of law's trans-cendence.

THE EVOCATION OF MYTH

Auden once asserted law's mythic singularity and gently remon-strated against identifying 'Law with some other word' (Auden 1966: 155). Of the two great traditions of conceiving law that we have considered, one would reduce law to the word authority and the other to the word society. The attempt to erect a posited being or a secure empire for law relied on social attributes of law, only then mysteriously to separate law from those attributes and set it above them. No less mysteriously, the attempt to identify law in social terms persistently invoked and eventually succumbed to law's distinct identity. Yet social accounts of law also persisted in their claim to be foundational of law. Law transcends society yet it is of society. The boundaries of law are inevitably and palpably set in relation to society but even in the face of the overwhelming evidence of law's social limits, popular belief in its transcendent efficacy persists (see e.g. Sarat 1990). This is not a matter of inconsistency or delusion. It is, as I will show in chapters 3 and 4, a matter of myth.

An Occidental encyclopaedia should presumably not be mute in uncovering the ground shared by these different perceptions of law. But where can we find an appropriate entry? 'Myth' would once have provided at least 'some god endowed with contradictory attributes' who could mediate between and encompass law's transcendent and terrestrial existences and render the common ground between them eloquent with sacred meaning (Lévi-Strauss 1968: 227). And there are indeed qualities of law which are also those of a god, at least one of a Christian persuasion. Law operates in a social world yet exists separate from and dominant over it. Law can relate integrally to that world without being existentially exhausted in the relation. It provides a principle and point of transcendent order and unity for the diversity of social relations and this as a matter of its own innate force (cf. Derrida 1990). It can transcend yet be in time to the effect that 'law is a presence which implies the totality of its history' (Goodrich and Hachamovitch 1991: 174). It successfully demands allegiance, not just to all that it was or is but also to all that it will be. The list could go on and, in later chapters, it will, but this is enough to show that here is a mystery.

Modern secular law takes identity in the rejection of transcendence: how can it sustain these deific qualities whilst rejecting transcendence? Law can no longer be elevated explicitly in terms of transcendent being – in terms such as those of divine or natural law. Its transcendent qualities are not and cannot be accommodated positively in terms of what law is. Perhaps they can be accommodated negatively in terms of what law is not. After all, 'the essence of this Law is that it has no essence' (Carty 1990: 6) – something which tends to be confirmed in the infinity of jurisprudential contests over what law is. Thus modern law emerges, in a negative exaltation, as universal in opposition to the particular, as unified in opposition to the diverse, as omnicompetent in contrast to the incompetent, and as controlling of what has to be controlled. (This list also will be extended later.) Law is imbued with this negative transcendence in its own myth of origin where it is imperiously set against certain 'others' who concentrate the qualities it opposes. Such others are themselves creatures of an Occidental mythology, a mythology which denies its own foundation by consigning myth in general to the world of these others. This compounded negation of myth does not mean that the mythology operative in the West is qualitatively different to that attributed to these benighted others. The two types of myth are, as I show in the next chapter, the same. The West's mythology against myth has all the characteristics it would locate in some savage mythology but it cannot recognize these characteristics as its own. The ground remains necessarily mute. Borges's alluring entry in the Chinese encyclopaedia combined with 'our' ignorance of the basis of his classification becomes a reflection of our own condition.

That is something of a premature conclusion to the chapter, but before leaving it I must consider the significant psychoanalytic search for myth in law. This search also entails a mute ground, some secret or mystery which is elusive yet informs law's uniform identity and transcendent capacities (e.g. Lenoble and Ost 1980:

50, 110, 227–9; 1986: 537, 543). It is law's authority, and the supposed vacuity of this authority, that especially provokes perception of some myth sustaining it (Goodrich 1990: chapter 6; see also Smith 1983: 237). Perhaps the most influential discovery of myth in law is made by Legendre who both proffers a psychoanalytical rendition of the myth yet maintains its ineluctable mystery (Legendre 1974, 1976).

The legal branch of the psychoanalytic study of myth has tended to concentrate narrowly on the dominance of the father. 'The legal paradigm is the will of the father' (Smith 1984: 245; cf. Duxbury 1990) – a father whose dominance seems more extensive than any envisaged by the most fervent Freudian. (On his death, the mythic lawgiver is mocked by Auden – or we are mocked in our dependence on him – as 'Our lost dad, Our colossal father' (Auden 1948: 98).) Legendre's refinement of this position proceeds by way of Freud and, as Duxbury emphasizes, by way of Lacan (Duxbury 1989). He effects a shift from a Law which in psychoanalytic terms orders the unconscious, and a shift from the Father as the figure of authority representing that Law, to equivalent figures inhabiting the legal terrain. The mythical figure of the Father imbues law with authority and unity by entering and lending force to law's mundane existence: but myth in law is not exhausted by this process and maintains a surpassing being into which law is elevated (Legendre 1974: 102; see also Lenoble and Ost 1980: 223, 1986: 537). In all, this seems to be less a matter of psychoanalysis explaining myth and more one of myth being enhanced by psychoanalysis. There remains an ultimate and irreducible mystery in the myth of law which calls for a particular psychological state of creative belief on the part of its adherents (Duxbury 1989: 93–4). People are subjected to law through their own construction of belief in a myth of law's authority. The surpassing nature of mystery would seem to accord with Legendre's elevation of myth as a poetic and aesthetic dimension of life which has been lost (see Goodrich 1990: chapter 8).

In some ways, I will adopt this account of myth. To the extent that it identifies a necessity for myth in law, I am happily in agreement with it. My agreement with its reliance on certain psychological states located in the unconscious or in conscious belief is more ambivalent, since I locate these states within a myth of modernity. And, finally, my seeing myth in terms of modernity does not fit the identification of myth with a world we have lost.

11

There is scope for oblique agreement here because I do have to recognize the explicit negation of myth in modernity, but that negation, as I show in the next chapter, is itself part of the myth of modernity.

I will resume the conclusion to this chapter. Having now evoked myth in law, I will concentrate in the next chapter on myth itself, before returning it to law in the following chapter 3 where law's mythic origin is traced. After providing a picture of pre-modern myth, I will show how myth now exists despite and because of its denial in modernity. The concern with denial and negation is then developed so as to found an account in chapter 3 of law as itself coming into being in modern myths of origin.

2

MYTH AND MODERNITY

I carry in my world that flourishes the worlds that have failed.

(Tagore 1926: 31)

GENESIS

In beginning *Homo Academicus*, Bourdieu counsels himself in these terms:

> The sociologist who chooses to study his own world in its nearest and most familiar aspects should not, as the ethnologist would, domesticate the exotic, but, if I may venture the expression, exoticize the domestic, through a break with his initial relation of intimacy with the mode of life and thought which remain opaque to him because they are too familiar.
>
> (Bourdieu 1988: xi)

If the existential claims of a world are more plausibly encompassing, such as those of the West and not just its academic microcosm, there are obvious difficulties about making this break. There is nowhere for an inhabitant of that world to stand apart. To claim a resolute and surpassing theoretical stance generated from within this world is the most common expedient. But this expedient is contrary to the whole argument of the present work. An enjoyable if no less fraught alternative could be to resort to another culture and, in that borrowed perspective, belabour the straitened epistemology of the West. My perspective, rather, seeks to subvert Western rationalities from within by heightening the contradictions and suppressions involved in their construction. It is an attempt at internal decolonization.

13

So, in this book, to 'exoticize the domestic', I look first at the Western domestic account of the exotic. I then show that such an exotic is integral to this realm of the domestic but also denied by it. Accounts of myth in Western scholarship present foundational forms of thought and belief that, so we are told, characterize non-Western 'others' and the pre-modern West. This is a presentation supposedly and basically contrasting with the way we are now. After analysing such accounts in this chapter, I devote the rest of it to the ways in which they are supposed to differ from Western modernity and to the beginnings of a reversal of that perspective. In those beginnings, I trace lineaments of myth in modernity and this becomes a prelude to the rest of the book.

Since modernity is opposed to myth, denying the relevance of myth to itself, there is an initial problem of how coherently to represent these accounts of myth in modern terms. Apart from the deeply contested coherence provided in particular intellectual fields – sociological functionalism, psychoanalysis and structuralism being the leading contenders this century – there is little that holds together the modern study of myth. Things considered of the essence in one account of myth will be completely lacking in another. In all, the modern study of myth comprises fairly constant but almost disjoint components of myth which seem to come together like a fugue whose harmonic impetus is not explicit in it. I do argue that myth is a suppressed dimension of modernity and I see its components finding a specific coherence in law as myth. That still leaves the problem of how initially to present these components of myth. Would that it were possible to erect a palindromic chapter in which the end point, where these components start to come together in modern myth, could be read back to this beginning. For the present, I will deal with the problem by briefly illustrating these components in particular myths and hope that compression will substitute for coherence as a guide to the rest of the chapter.

I start with an instance of the familiarly exotic and summarize that origin myth of the Hebrews recounted in chapter 1 of *Genesis*, supplemented by parts of that and other books of Moses. Before the beginning, as it were, 'the earth was without form and void: and darkness was upon the face of the deep'. There is a god (to whom we should deny singularity given the diversity of deities, and of their genders, evoked in the gnostic gospels) who creates light and divides the light from the darkness. 'And God called the light

Day, and the darkness he called Night'. The god continues in this process of division and classification as 'he' goes about creating the earth, the seas, the stars and so on. He also 'made the firmament, and divided the waters which were under the firmament from the waters which were above the firmament . . . . And God called the firmament Heaven.' Earth and the seas brought forth a variety of plants and animals 'after their kind'. Finally, the god made 'man in our image and after our likeness' and gave man dominion over all the other creatures and the mandate to subdue the earth. In another origin myth from chapter 2 of *Genesis* we learn that the god formed the first man, Adam, 'of the dust of the ground . . . and whatsoever Adam called every living creature, that was the name thereof'. The story does, of course, go on. It is from a collection of myths that guided a group of people who saw themselves as chosen by the god. The legendary author of the story, as we learn from Deuteronomy, brought the law for a new society from heaven to earth in the descent from Mount Sinai.

I will take one other example of a myth, one which appears in many respects to be close to the first, but the correspondence is not forced. It is a myth of an Aboriginal group in what is now called Australia:

> The truth is, of course, that my own people, the Riratjingu, are descended from the great Djankawu who came from the island of Baralku far across the sea. Our spirits return to Baralku when we die. Djankawu came in his canoe with his two sisters, following the morning star which guided them to the shores of Yelangbara on the eastern coast of Arnhem Land. They walked far across the country following the rain clouds. When they wanted water they plunged their digging stick into the ground and fresh water flowed. From them we learnt the names of all the creatures on the land and they taught us all our Law.
>
> (Isaacs 1980: 5)

From and somewhat around these stories, we can extract components of myth. The stories deal with origins and identity, and in particular here with the origins and identity of a group or a people. With the Aboriginal story this is their 'Dreaming'. They cannot use, nor can this be used as, another group's Dreaming. With *Genesis*, I have merely presented the opening of a more prolix and more familiar account of origins and identity. The myth often

15

claims, or is the basis for claiming, an exclusive humanity or at least a superiority for the group. Origins are located in a special way. The point of origin is sacred – set apart, made transcendent and beyond encompassing in profane experience. The god in the firmament of Heaven provides one instance and the great Djankawu from the island of Baralku provides another. This origin, as with the god of *Genesis*, is usually a source of continuing creation or influence. Such a self-generating, sacred force imposes and sustains an order from above. The ability to do this is often transferred in part to agents such as the first man made in the image of the god. Forces stand separately or apart from and act on that which is more inert or beneath them. Such powers of creation and domination are frequently held to be concentrated in some central point, just as Eden was the centre of the world. Agents, forces and centres are connected with the profane world but they partake of and take their reality from the sacred. They mediate between the two realms. In *Genesis* man is made from dust yet in the image of the god. The culture hero Djankawu and his two sisters come from the sacred island of origin to live in and shape the land.

Such mediations locate the profane, mortal world within the sacred, providing members of the group with guidance and orientation to a reality which is perceived and lived through myth. Djankawu and his sisters discover and mark out the primal terrain, they name the creatures and they taught us all our Law. *Genesis* maps out a world in which the man is given the power to name. *Genesis* itself is part of a collection of myths containing the god's message, a guide to life encapsulated in the Law which Moses carries from heaven to earth. Such mediations transcend what would otherwise be the insuperable limits and contradictions of the profane world. They connect people with ultimate origins and ultimate identity, with the source and foundational force of all that is. Myth both sets the limits of the world, of what can be meant and done, and transcends these limits in its relation to the sacred. The contradictions exist within the myth, but they are mediated by it – by the coherence or conduct of the mythic story or simply through obfuscation such as, for example, through placing contradictory elements in distinct but related myths. It is this relation between myths which I cannot cover in an account illustrated by isolated examples. This is a relation of dependence of a myth on other myths for the revelation of its 'full' meaning. Here I will just provide a reference, following up one of my examples, to Leach's dazzling analysis of 'Genesis as myth' (Leach 1969). Having presented what I hope is an adequate, short illustration of the components of myth I will now expand on it.

THE MYTH OF MYTH

'Myth' is a modern entrant into the English language. As such, it contrasts negatively with history and science, forms commonly said to have displaced it – myth predominantly imports 'what could not really exist or have happened' (see Williams 1983: 211–12). Myth is either false or an oblique, inadequate presentation of something that is more true than it can be. Those who believe in myth, whether ancients or primitives, are credulous and uninventive. Whether they were or are is not part of my concern here but this view of them is indicative of a certain Western incapacity which becomes significant for the argument later in this chapter. With Western notions of the indivisibility of truth, myth is inevitably found wanting. In his analysis of myths of virgin birth, Leach remarks that 'the anthropologist's belief in the ignorance of his primitive contemporaries shows an astonishing resilience in the face of adverse evidence' (Leach 1969: 85). Debates about whether the Trobriand Islanders, for example, believed that the male was a dispensable element in procreation could have been refined in Malinowski's observation that 'the natives distinguish definitely between myth and historic account' (Malinowski 1961: 299). Leach finds that among such 'primitive contemporaries . . . doctrines about the possibility of conception taking place without male insemination do not stem from innocence and ignorance: on the contrary they are consistent with theological argument of the greatest subtlety' (Leach 1969: 85–6). He pours effective scorn on Frazer, of *The Golden Bough* (1914), who would hold such 'magic' views in contempt yet 'offer . . . no objection to the nightly recital of Latin grace in Trinity College Hall' (Leach 1969: 92). There are, however, exceptions to the negative view of myth. Some, whilst recognising the decline or demise of myth, would yet discern truths in myth and would advocate its recognition or revival, or they engage in varieties of deliberate mythopoeia. The analysis of dreams in depth psychology provides the most significant recent source of these attempts.

I will arrange the rest of this analysis of the modern study of

17

myth around two broad perspectives brought to bear on it. One could be called experiential and viewed in terms of an inter- pretative or phenomenological sociology. It looks at myth as it may be for those who adhere to it. The other is usually and simply called sociological but it is a particular type of sociology, one which attempts to provide objective explanations of myth. I will consider each in turn.

In the experiential approach, myth is seen as a sacred story. Eliade is a leading exponent:

> We are at last beginning to know and understand the value of the myth, as it has been elaborated in 'primitive' and archaic societies – that is, among those groups of mankind where the myth happens to be the very foundation of social life and culture. Now, one fact strikes us immediately: in such societies the myth is thought to express the *absolute truth*, because it narrates a *sacred history*; that is, a transhuman revelation which took place at the dawn of the Great Time, in the holy time of the beginnings (*in illo tempore*). Being *real* and *sacred*, the myth becomes exemplary, and consequently *repeatable*, for it serves as a model, and by the same token as a justification, for all human actions. In other words, a myth is a *true history* of what came to pass at the beginning of Time, and one which provides the pattern for human behaviour. In *imitating* the exemplary acts of a god or of a mythic hero, or simply by recounting their adventures, the man of an archaic society detaches himself from profane time and magically re-enters the Great Time, the sacred time.
>
> (Eliade 1968: 23 – his emphasis)

In a comprehensive survey of extant approaches to the study of myth, what Cohen finds invariant is the idea of myth as a sacred narrative of origins and transformation (Cohen 1969: 337). This quality of the sacred typifies the origins themselves. The sacred- ness of myth and origins consists in their being set apart and held sacrosanct or inviolable. The origins come from another realm, a sacred realm beyond the natural and beyond the profane. Origins provide a foundation and ultimate reference: 'In the beginning was the Word, and the Word was with God, and the Word was God' (John 1:1). (Formative force and original creative power are often put in terms connoting speech.) The foundation as ultimate under lies and grounds all else – 'God of God, Light of Light, true

God of true God' (The Nicene Creed). It is not knowable or fully knowable. It is often rendered as persistent and pervasive. Origins are a creation and the beginnings of a continued creative and assertive force. In Christian mythology there is the idea of the sovereign creator – the King of Kings, the Lord of Lords – who rules over and maintains the universe in accordance with his laws. The creative force acts on undifferentiated, formless, limitless and nocturnal chaos. It brings forth and forms, or makes manifest, the cosmos and the world, including the group whose origin is being recounted. The story will sustain this creative impetus into something of a present with its telling of how things came and continued to be as they are, including the place – the being and the belonging – of the group and its members in the world and the cosmos. Typically, it will account for the relations within the group and relations between the group and others. It will tell of the relations people have with time and the course of nature, with animals and plants. It will relate different people to different cultural activities – cooking, material production, ritual. These various categories of relations will connect integrally and provide an elaborate guide to life.

The plane of myth is not, then, confined to the sacred. As it is so often put, 'myths describe the . . . breakthrough of the sacred . . . into the world' (Eliade 1963: 6). It is such a 'breakthrough of the sacred that really *establishes* the world' – and establishes the world as real – including 'man himself' as 'a mortal, sexed and cultural being' (Eliade 1963: 6 – his emphasis). The sacred 'renders human existence possible – prevents it, that is, from regression to the level of zoological existence' (Eliade 1968: 19). It is by partaking in the sacred that persons and things become real. The sacred in myth transfigures the profane, giving it form, efficacy and validity:

> Evidently, for the archaic mentality, reality manifests itself as force, effectiveness, and duration. Hence the outstanding reality is the sacred: for only the sacred *is* in an absolute fashion, acts effectively, creates things and makes them endure. The innumerable gestures of consecration – of tracts and territories, of objects, of men, etc. – reveal the primitive's obsession with the real, his thirst for being.
>
> (Eliade 1965: 11 – his emphasis)

To take an example, Eliade sets a scene of 'wild, uncultivated

19

regions and the like' which in myths 'are assimilated to chaos; they
. . . participate in the undifferentiated, formless modality of pre-
creation' (Eliade 1965: 9). Onto this scene enter original colonists:

> Their enterprise was for them only the repetition of a prim-
> ordial act: the transformation of chaos into cosmos by the
> divine act of Creation. By cultivating the desert soil, they in
> fact repeated the act of the gods, [or civilizing heroes] who
> organized chaos by giving it forms and norms. Better still, a
> territorial conquest does not become real until after – more
> precisely, through – the ritual of taking possession, which is
> only a copy of the primordial act of the Creation of the
> World.
>
> (Eliade 1965: 10)

So, although the transcendent, sacred realm and an operative
reality are separable, they are ultimately identified with each other.
Putting it in the negative vein, myth is said to confuse the ideal and
the real (e.g. Bidney 1958: 11). Hence, as it is often and dubiously
said, primitives engaging in magic ritual do not distinguish between reality and the effect of the ritual: the world has in reality
survived, the crops have in reality grown because the correct rituals
were performed. 'Nature is thought to yield nothing without cere-
monies' (Bidney 1958: 9). Shamanistic dances, divination and
garden magic do not simply imitate the original, exemplary acts of
a god or hero. The invocation of these acts is an identification with
them, their presencing and reiteration, and an exercise of their
power and force. Thus, myth provides 'a warrant of magical efficiency' and the impotence of the here and now is transcended
(Malinowski 1932: 455). Myth operates on and in the here and
now, conferring force and meaning on it. A law, for example, is
effective because of its correspondence to a transcendent model or
origin. For Barthes, the operative model of meaning in 'bourgeois'
society becomes effective mythically in that historical meaning is
elevated to a plane of the natural as universal (Barthes 1973: 129).

The relationship people have with myth is 'based on use'
(Barthes 1973: 144). Myth is 'the expression of a *mode of being in the
world*' (Eliade 1968: 124 – his emphasis). Myth is not only an
expression, however. It imperatively guides action and establishes
patterns of behaviour. This guidance is not merely subordinating.
People employ it, as I have just indicated, to exert control in the
here and now. For example, to know the origin of the thing is to

control it (Eliade 1963: 18). Claims are thus upheld and rights legitimated. Myth is 'a hard-worked active force . . . a pragmatic charter' (Malinowski 1954: 101).

This necessary usability is accompanied by contradictory characteristics of myth. These could be approached obliquely through the question of whether myth is poetic. It is often said to be, usually in the setting of worlds we have lost but must regain, in tales of regret and resurrection. For Lévi-Strauss, however, when considering the problem of translation:

> Poetry is a kind of speech which cannot be translated except at the cost of serious distortions; whereas the mythical value of the myth is preserved even through the worst translation. Myth is language, functioning on an especially high level where meaning succeeds practically at 'taking off' from the linguistic ground on which it keeps on rolling.
>
> (Lévi-Strauss 1968: 210)

Barthes would see myth and poetry in opposition but he would grant to 'classical poetry' the status of 'a strongly mythical system, since it imposes on the meaning one extra signified, which is *regularity*' (Barthes 1973: 133 – his emphasis).

Such elements of regularity and general accessibility of meaning are reflected in the narrative quality of myth. The narrative form makes contents of myth explicit and tangible. Whilst narrative and its exact rendition may seem essential for the usability of myth in some societies, its significance and its necessity for myth in general have been questioned. For Lévi-Strauss the 'truth' of a myth is found in its combination with other myths (Lévi-Strauss 1968: chapter XI). Each myth is a fragment and what counts is a collection of myths and the structured connection between them. Narrative in this view is secondary – a mode of holding configurations of meaning together. Other means, it could be added, would do as well. Even if a narrative were essential for the effectiveness of myth in oral cultures, need it be so in modern, literate ones with intense and diverse modes of preserving and communicating information? Might not the alleged loss of myth along with modernity, so often equated with the loss of a poetic dimension, be but the loss of a dispensable mode of its rendition? Be all this as it may, I will also argue towards the end of this chapter that narrative is a characteristic, if not invariable, feature of modern Western mythology.

21

Ritual is another mode of locating myth in experience, of making myth accessible, regular and, in short, usable. It will often overlap with narrative since the telling of a myth can be a ritual or can take place on a ritual occasion. The ritual preparation and application of a medicinal cure, for example, will often be accompanied by the recitation of the myth of its origin in the time of the beginning. Rituals are evocations and instanciations of myth, tangible assertions of the natural order – of order made natural. The performance of ritual is often in the hands of specialists – of shamans, diviners, sorcerers and various practitioners of magic. The same can be the case in the guarding and transmitting of mythic knowledge: 'he who recites the myths has had to prove his vocation and receive instruction from the old masters' (Eliade 1963: 145).

Here is the beginning of a paradox in the usability of myth. Myth as an accessible and regular mode of being in the world, as a mode of making the deepest truths of life generally operative, stands in contrast to myth as the preserve of storytellers and performers of ritual (see e.g. Davidson 1990). To explore this paradox, I return to the non-poetic nature of myth and to the remove between language and the meaning of myth. I will do so in the company of Maurice Bloch along with his essay on 'Symbols, Song, Dance and Features of Articulation' (Bloch 1974). Ritual entails 'a formalization of language', formalized speech and singing, formalized dance (Bloch 1974: 57–8, 72). 'Ritual is an occasion where syntactic and other linguistic freedoms are reduced because ritual makes special uses of language: characteristically stylised speech and singing' (Bloch 1974: 56). Language in such situations has a certain '"set apart" character' and the participants thus come to see ritual 'as being outside themselves' and 'invariant' (Bloch 1974: 56, 68). 'The reason for this dramatic impoverishment in linguistic choice is the fantastic creativity potential of natural language', including, doubtless, its potential to destroy the identity of the ritual (Bloch 1974: 61). Language thence becomes distinct, bounded and subject to appropriation by authority. It becomes 'a form of power or coercion' (Bloch 1974: 60). There is restriction on what can be said and on responses to what can be said but it cannot be that authority and restriction rule out general participation in ritual. The ultimate reach of the paradox of formalization is – borrowing here Legendre's notion of 'solemnisation' – that it 'consists in creating the distance necessary for the subject to enter discourse and equally in exempting the subject from having to speak on his own account' (see Goodrich 1990: 279). This account of ritual and language has now taken us near domains to which an objective sociology would lay claim, and I now consider it.

The interpretative approach is frequently advanced in false modesty as the alternative to a hubristic sociology but the two approaches can overlap even in their own terms. No matter how effective objective observers may be, the observed may be sufficiently acute to share insights with them. In Malinowski's eyes, the Trobriand Islanders could be good sociologists (see e.g. Malinowski 1961: 303). The outside observer would, however, claim to go further than the adherents of myth were able to go. If, for example, we take the classic Durkheimian position, we could say that a myth expresses and maintains social solidarity. The observer knows this function in a way that is more extensive, more complete than the local knowledge of the observed who do not see as fully how myths affect them. This is basic stuff and little more than an echo of a fundamental debate in the social sciences, to take it no further than that. Here, I am merely concerned to isolate the objective stance as part of components of myth created in Western knowledge.

In the objective vision, followers of myth live in a limited world which objectivity inclusively encompasses and understands. This world is one which can only be fully known from the outside, a world within which things can never be what they seem. It is a world which may have its constrained rationalities, but it is ultimately knowable only through scientific reason, or some such (see e.g. Evans-Pritchard 1937: chapter 4). The very limits of this world are discernible in myth. Cohen thus summarizes 'Malinowski's incomparable description and analysis':

> Malinowski's Trobrianders are business-like men, very much of this world; and if they believe stories about original witches it is because like all men, they run up against the limits of reason and fact. To legitimate their institutions they need some sort of charter which is beyond fact, beyond reason and refers to events beyond memory and ordinary time. The rules which govern everyday life are always, in some respects and to some extent, in doubt: real history, real patterns of migration and settlement, real claims to property and power, always

23

THE MYTHOLOGY OF MODERN LAW

> involve inconsistencies and irreconcilable demands: myths,
> in recounting the events of an invented or partly-invented
> past, resolve these inconsistencies and affirm one set of
> claims as against another. The introduction of imaginary
> events takes the point of origin out of the realm of memory:
> and the introduction of unreal events gives the story a quality
> which transcends the mundane.
>
> (Cohen 1969: 344)

The reality of myth is always something else, somewhere else. If a
Trobriand myth is ostensibly about flying witches, it is really about
clan rights: if it is ostensibly about original people emerging from
holes in the ground, it is really about territorial rights: if it is
ostensibly about the origins of a spell, it is really about legitimating
otherwise unfounded magical claims. Myths set limits by 'blocking
off explanation' of things as they really may, or may not be: in this
way they are 'means for legitimating social practices' (Cohen 1969:
351). Their efficacy in blocking off explanation and legitimating
social practices 'would be enhanced by their use of symbolism
which galvanised the deepest commitments and feelings of rever-
ence and sacredness, and by use of style, which presents a dramatic
tension between opposed objects or forces which is somehow
resolved' (Cohen 1969: 351). Myth is, in Marx's phrase, 'a reversed
world': it is a reflection of those social practices which it is
fantastically credited with creating (see Marx and Engels 1957:
41–2). The world of myth is, then, a world of limits which captures
those within it. Beyond those limits there is for those captives the
unknown or the dimly known, including that chaos or primal
matter out of which were fashioned what is and what is known.
That which is beyond those limits pertains to the gods, to fate, to
the nature of things, even if the primitive or the ancient may see in
these domains prospects of an expansive participation in the
sacred and the numinomus – prospects of having life more abundantly (John 10: 10).

Having discovered myth as limits, the objective approach
locates its defining function in mediating contradiction resulting
from those limits. Myth is about the resolution of inconsistencies,
the resolution of opposition (Cohen 1969: 344, 351). For Lévi-
Strauss 'myth serves to provide an apparent resolution, or
"mediation", of problems which are by their very nature incapable
of any final resolution' (Leach 1969: 54). I will use 'mediation' to

connote a reconciling of opposites – life and death, light and dark, us and them, legitimate and illegitimate. Resolution or apparent resolution is not necessarily involved since myth will often effect a reconciliation through obfuscation rather than resolution. As Lévi-Strauss would recognize: 'the repetitions and prevarications of mythology so fog the issue that irresolvable logical inconsistencies are lost sight of even when they are openly expressed' (Leach 1974: 58). Myth also creates contradictions which it then mediates. Being of a transcendent realm, it will at least create contradictions with the mundane. For example, the domination of one group over another, changing and uncertain as it is in time, is mythically elevated to the timeless; the opposition between the temporal and the eternal is then mediated by giving the domination a divine origin. Something less than strict reconciliation is also involved where myth, as is often the case, simply restates contradiction in another plane.

Indeed, the main mode of mediation is the transfer of contradiction to some other, intractable plane – to the realm of gods, fate, nature or complete virtue. The Ascension of Christ is close to an analogue of the process. A contradiction between his human and divine nature is ultimately resolved through his human body being taken up into and becoming part of the divine. Myth, as we saw when considering the interpretative perspective, involves things of this world taking on a transcendent and exemplary reality through their participation in the sacred and it is this participation which gives the real its form and its force. A drab objectivity would reverse that world and see the timeless and sacred as an expedient reflection and mollifying avoidance of contradiction within the inescapably mundane.

Lévi-Strauss greatly extends the range of mediating transformations in myth, even if it can be unclear how the resulting connections are made. Thus, in *The Raw and the Cooked*, he explores the myths of certain Indian groups in Brazil dealing with the origin of cooking (Lévi-Strauss 1986). Cooking, as the transformation of the raw, is connected with the transformation of nature into culture. The raw and the rotten mark a return to nature. Such a set of relations in complex ways connects a great many other things including, to borrow a summary from Cohen, 'themes of cosanguinity, affinity, incest and its prohibitions, exogamy, inclusion, exclusion, and so on' (Cohen 1969: 347). 'The true constituent units of a myth are not the isolated relations but *bundles of such relations*, and it is only as bundles that these relations can be put to use and combined so as to produce a meaning' (Lévi-Strauss 1968: 211 – his emphasis).

Figures are created in myth mediating between the diverse planes or sites in opposition. Heroes or monsters straddling the chaos and order will often have a parent who is divine. Thus Gilgamesh of Mesopotamian myth was two-thirds divine and one-third human. The Church is of this earth but also Christ's mystical body. A city will be the centre of the world and the meeting point of heaven and earth. Honey comes from the wild but it is collected and used in cooking and so marks a mediation between nature and culture (Lévi-Strauss 1987: 43–4). The trickster figure is another common mediator. The raven and the coyote in many North American Indian myths are instances of such figures. As carrion-eating they are like beasts of prey in eating animals but they are like producers of food plants in not killing what they eat. Thence, they mediate in numerous and complex ways between agriculture and hunting and between life and death (see Lévi-Strauss 1968: 224–5). The trickster, says Lévi-Strauss, like all mediating figures, 'must retain something of that duality' it mediates, 'namely an ambiguous and equivocal character' (Lévi-Strauss 1968: 226). Mediating figures are an instance of the malleability and the protean – Proteus being another example – nature of myth. Everything is possible with myth (Leach 1974: 87). Anything can become anything else. Mythic heroes can be all-powerful or all-knowing. Christ was of the Godhead. Gilgamesh found out all things and experienced everything. The labile character of myth extends to the way it changes in time. To extract the meaning of the myth, as Lévi- Strauss has shown, it must be taken to include all its versions or transformations (Lévi-Strauss 1986: 1–14). What is more, myth would seem to retain an openness or something short of completeness: myths are 'interminable' (Lévi-Strauss 1986: 6). Myths are also 'mutually transformational' and the object of investigation for the study of myth is a resulting 'mythical field' (Lévi-Strauss 1987: 55). Every myth is 'one of a complex and . . . any pattern which occurs in one myth will recur, in the same or other variations, in another part of the complex' (Leach 1969: 22). To extract the meaning of myth and to identify the full range of its mediations, myth has to be placed integrally in the mythical field: 'the sum of what all the myths say is not expressly said by any of them' (Leach 1974: 71–2). In some of these relations myths will be synonymous or supportive, in others opposed. Hence one has to consider a 'complex' or 'set' of such myths in the Bible so as to 'resolve' the contradiction between the rule requiring Jewish endogamy and the frequency of exogamy (Leach 1969: 22, 40).

THE DENIGRATION OF MYTH

Such a sociology in its claim to encompass myth, as something essentially different to itself, belongs to a tradition of Western thought that pre-dates its own invention. In modern times, from at least the eighteenth century, mythology has been relegated to the fabulous and the false in contrast to reality and to its forms in science and history which were launched on an unbounded quest for truth. This limitless and constantly critical quest stood in opposition to the constrained fixity and set superstition of mythology. For Adorno and Horkheimer, 'the program of the Enlightenment was the disenchantment of the world: the dissolution of myth and the substitution of knowledge for fancy' (Adorno and Horkheimer 1979: 3). And 'the opposition of enlightenment to myth is expressed in the opposition of the . . . individual ego to multifarious fate' (Adorno and Horkheimer 1979: 46). It was the liberated sovereign subject of Enlightenment who would dare to know and dare not to remain secure within the ignorance and delusion of the mythic. Further, 'in the anticipatory identification of the wholly conceived . . . world with truth, enlightenment intends to secure itself against the return of the mythic' (Adorno and Horkheimer 1979: 25).

The division between myth and truth can be illustrated in a brief overview of history and myth. Malinowski, with some gentle envy, thus describes the belief behind Trobriand myths:

> They have no idea of what could be called the evolution of the world or the evolution of society; that is, they do not look back towards a series of successive changes, which happened in nature or in humanity, as we do. We, in our religious and scientific outlook alike, know that earth ages and that humanity ages, and we think of both in these terms; for them, both are eternally the same, eternally youthful.
>
> (Malinowski 1961: 301)

The distinction is put in many ways. One of the more vivid is the division between 'cold' and 'hot' societies:

27

> Cold societies are those that seem to annul by special institutions the effects of historical factors on their equilibrium and continuity and hot societies are those that internalise the historical process and make it the moving power of their development.
>
> (Munz 1973: ix)

Eliade's theme in *The Myth of the Eternal Return* is that 'historical man' makes himself in history but 'archaic man' seeks to escape 'the terror of history' through self-subjection to fixed myth: in this 'refusal to accept himself as a historical being' time and the unusual are denied value (Eliade 1965: ix, 85–6). Myth, as the ultimate reality for archaic man, provides a charter for doing things forever in the unvarying repetition of what is originally formulated – in an eternal return. Myth 'reveals something as having been *fully manifested*, and this manifestation is at the same time *exemplary*' in its being a foundation and guide for human behaviour (Eliade 1968: 16 – his emphasis).

Myth is thus modernity's pre-creation. Just as chaos is the pre-creation and antithesis of myth, so myth precedes and is negated by modernity. Modernity is what myth is not. The perception of myth as illusion and the means of finding true foundations of existence come with 'the advance of reason and self-conscious reflection' (Bidney 1958: 21), an advance inextricable with that of the autonomous individual as the locus of universal being, as the condensation of humanity. This is not an achieved state. It is constantly to be achieved in a process of becoming which locates all that was as a prelude to and increment towards all that will be. This becoming is antithetical to the fixed being of myth.

Such an identity through becoming does not entail an invariant rejection of myth. Here we must inevitably talk of Greeks and distinctions. The Greeks, like the primitives: 'had their roots in the primeval slime . . . but what the myths show is how high they had risen above the ancient filth and fierceness by the time we have any knowledge of them. Only a few traces of that time are to be found in the stories' (Hamilton 1953: 14). These myths are absorbed into the Western tradition as part of the progressive story of transcendence beyond myth, a transcendence intimated by the pre-Socratic philosophers in their elevation of 'science' and their pitting of *logos* against *mythos* (Cornford 1932) – but the sharpness and significance of the division are debated (cf. Cornford 1957).

Euhemerus in the third century BC even provides a distanced sociological perspective on myth. Such presentiments and developments were beyond the monotonous primitives who remained an unredeemed limiting case in the pre-creation of modernity. Their mythic world enduringly contrasts with that of ancient Greece:

> Nothing is clearer than the fact that primitive man, whether in New Guinea today or eons ago in the prehistoric wilderness, is not and never has been a creature who peoples his world with bright fancies and lovely visions. Horrors lurked in the primeval forest, not nymphs and naiads. Terror lived there, with its close attendant Magic.
>
> (Hamilton 1953: 14)

And so on. If something a little more academically exalted is wanted, there is Leslie A. White's still influential *The Evolution of Culture* in which we learn that the knowledge possessed by 'primitive peoples' is not 'naturalistic, genuine knowledge' but 'the pseudo knowledge of mythology' which can involve identification with 'subhuman species' (White 1959: 265, 274). There is, of course, much more of this sort of thing and I will deal with it more systematically in the next two chapters. This is only a general idea for this general account of myth. And there are exceptions to the prevalent denigration of myth. Some have treated myth positively as itself having universal contents, but these enterprises have remained Eurocentric. The structural analyses of myth as patterns of the mind advanced by Lévi-Strauss depend on oppositions, such as that between nature and culture, which are at least questionable in their claims to universality. Taking another immensely influential instance of recent times, there could be scepticism about what 'collective' is involved in Jung's notion of the 'collective unconscious' as a repository of universal mythic themes (see Fanon 1967: 190–1).

THE PERFECTION OF MYTH

Denigrated myth becomes the obverse of a Western world. This was a newly created world set against a past or passing world of mythic tradition – 'the woof of time is every instant broken, the track of generations effaced' (Tocqueville 1862: 119). It was a world that now took identity as the culmination yet negation of all

29

that preceded it (Marx 1973: 106). Such an identity is constantly recreated and sustained in opposition to certain 'others' who persist as embodiments of contrary worlds that have gone before. The primitive, to take a figure of the other, is uncontrolled, fickle, irresponsible, of nature, and so on. The European is disciplined, constant, self-responsible, of culture, and so on. But the other is not truly other (even assuming such a state were possible). It does not exist primarily or initially apart from its relation to a West which encompasses it. The other, in its uncivilized or pre-modern state, is a construct of the West (see e.g. Said 1985). A closure is thus effected. The West creates those others in simple opposition to which it is created. The closure is, in a Western perspective, impregnable in that the other cannot speak against it because of the West's arrogation to itself of truth as singular yet universal. The other is incorporated within that truth yet maintained as other and it cannot deny or disturb the rightness of its inert place within that truth. In this hopeless inadequacy, the other is unable to stand against the European's all-encompassing sufficiency. The European can, then, relate to the other without extending or revealing itself.

The argument can be made tangible in Goodrich's moving account of a recent case involving the Haida Indians who had attempted to prevent a logging company desecrating their ancestral land (Goodrich 1990: 179–84). The company operated under a licence given by the government of British Columbia. It brought an action seeking to uphold the licence and to obtain an injunction preventing further interference with logging by the Haida. The Indians wished to represent themselves and to speak in their own terms. The first response of the court to this desire was portentous. It consisted of attempts to persuade the Indians to employ legal representatives so as to bring themselves within the language and the mastery of the law. To this the Indian response was that 'the issue of our lands is too important to leave in the hands of lawyers who are unfamiliar with our people' (Goodrich 1990: 180). The court then adopted a seemingly liberal stance and accepted testimony which 'took the form of symbolic dress, mythologies, masks and totem poles as well as the legends, stories, poems, songs and other forms of interpretation that such art and mythology implied' (Goodrich 1990: 182–3). Such testimony told of the mythic origin of the Haida and of their identification with the land. The Haida also extended themselves to the European other by including evidence in Western terms about Haida customary law concerning dispute settlement and land claims. The judicial response was brutal in effect if not intent:

> Unreserved judgment was given by the court the day after argument ended. Justice McKay observed that the court would not normally have allowed argument of the political kind heard but that, in view of the fact that the Haida had no other arena available to them, he had been prepared to listen and generously recommended that a record of the evidence presented should be kept for posterity. The judgment itself was extremely brief. The evidence presented as the Haida title to and relationship with the islands was not legally relevant to the case being heard, which simply concerned interference with a valid logging licence.
>
> (Goodrich 1990: 183)

The argument of the Haida to be preserved for posterity was but 'a curiosity, a relic, a primitive remnant of a more savage past' (Goodrich 1990: 183). The attempt 'to speak for ourselves' was comprehensively negated – the court treated it as a charade, admitting it because there was 'no other arena available to them':

> The court would not compare mythologies, *it refused even to countenance the question of the 'other'*, because to do so would raise questions of its 'self', of the social and mythic construction of its own body, its social role and actions, its own clothes.
>
> (Goodrich 1990: 183 – his emphasis)

How, then, can we begin to locate myth where it is not, to find myth in its negation? We could look for remnants of myth, for so-called survivals. The dress and rituals of the law court are often seen in this way. But this is to cede the terrain before entering it. I will argue that myth in modernity is more typical and infinitely more extensive than a matter of survivals. Another approach would be to try and locate myth in disguise. Ideology looks a likely contender. It is often taken to include myth, among many other things (e.g. Feldman and Richardson 1972). It does involve something of a transcendence of the idea and some also see it as 'embodied within a specific set of material practices' (see Urry 1981: 3). These two characteristics, as we have seen, could be equated with significant dimensions of myth. Also, as I show later, there are more extensive parallels between myth and Lefort's notion of 'bourgeois ideology' (Lefort 1986: chapter 6). Still, I would want to sustain myth as distinct and as more specifically elaborated than ideology.

My approach, rather, will be to confront the supposed absence of myth in modernity, beginning with the help provided by Derrida in his 'White Mythology: Metaphor in the Text of Philosophy' (Derrida 1982: 207–71). Derrida takes a concern which could be seen as obscure in a couple of senses, a speculative concern with the metaphorical origins of Western metaphysics – and one which has long parallels in the study of myth (see e.g. Munz 1973). Metaphysical ideas, some would say, develop in their use through a progressive erasure or obscuring of their metaphorical content. In the ultimate meaning of the idea, metaphor is eliminated or relegated and its use can thence only be an aid or adornment in expressing the idea. Derrida proceeds to demonstrate the inescapability of metaphor. Expressions of the very attempt to eliminate metaphor are also found to be metaphorical in their force and origin. (Perhaps the very notion of metaphor itself suggests a pure meaning that precedes the addition of the compromising metaphorical element.) The outcome, as Derrida would derive it from Anatole France, is that:

> By an odd fate, the very metaphysicians who think to escape the world of appearances are constrained to live perpetually in allegory. A sorry lot of poets, they dim the colours of the ancient fables, and are themselves but gatherers of fables. They produce white mythology.
>
> (Derrida 1982: 213)

'White' here, it seems, is to be understood in two related senses. In one, white is an absence, devoid of colour, 'an anaemic mythology' (Derrida 1982: 213). The other sense of white connects with Derrida's constant engagement with the grounds and authority of Western knowledge:

> Metaphysics – the white mythology which reassembles and reflects the culture of the West; the white man takes his own mythology, Indo-European mythology, his own *logos*, that is the *mythos* of his idiom, for the universal form of that he must still wish to call Reason . . . . White mythology – metaphysics has erased within itself the fabulous scene that has produced

it, the scene that nevertheless remains active and stirring, inscribed in white ink, an invisible design covered over in the palimpsest.

(Derrida 1982: 213)

There are problems in a ready reliance on this as establishing a Western mythology. The simple equation of mythology with a metaphysics is hardly accurate or extensive enough for my concerns. Nor can myth be merely identified with metaphor, even if this were Derrida's intention. Myth is but one form of metaphor and to establish the inevitability of metaphor is not necessarily to establish the inevitability of myth or mythology. But I do draw on two things which Derrida does in relation to myth. First, he does posit terms that counterpoint the supposed absence of myth in modernity. White mythology corresponds to an anaemia or void, 'invisibly' yet inexorably and densely populated by that which was supposedly eliminated in its making. I will return often to this theme. Second, in making out his argument, Derrida does draw on metaphors with a strong mythic resonance. I will now consider some of these as illustrating mythic contents which I deal with later.

There are two broad types of metaphor Derrida draws on, both of which correspond to persistent and connected themes in his own thought – metaphors of foundation and force. First, there are varieties of philosophy's metaphorical 'foundation': 'what is fundamental corresponds to the desire for a firm and ultimate ground, a terrain to build on, the earth as the support of an artificial structure' (Derrida 1982: 224). Founding concepts have a force, 'their own metaphysical charge': 'the concept of the concept cannot not retain the gesture of mastery, taking and maintaining in the present, comprehending and grasping the thing as an object' (Derrida 1982: 224). Force operates in creative tensions and contradictions such as that between culture and nature or that between law and nature (Derrida 1982: 220, 226, 228). Force also has distinctness and sufficiency. To take only its form in light, the optic metaphor claims close to a sensory exclusiveness in Western theory (see Derrida 1982: 224; see also Foucault 1970). In light, I would add, there is comprehensive revelation; it evokes an undiminished origin and straight and unbroken paths in the pursuit of knowledge. With Descartes, 'prior to every determined presence, to every representative idea, natural light constitutes the very ether of thought and of its proper discourse' (see Derrida 1982: 267). Eventually, inevitably light takes on local habitation and a name delineated in one of Derrida's footnotes. Light travels, as Hegel helpfully reminds us, from East to West, coeval with 'the History of the World . . . , for Europe is absolutely the end of History' (see Derrida 1982: 269). In this History, light ultimately comes to reside within, to be encompassed by, the fully conscious individual of Europe who not only knows but also acts on and makes the world: 'by the close of day', says Hegel, 'man has erected a building constructed from his own inner Sun' (see Derrida 1982: 269). The colours of the ancient fables have not been much dimmed after all.

This individual is the great mythic figure of the modern age. Nietzsche revealed in the death God an absence of correspondence between the real and some ordering, transcendent realm. For 'us' who have killed God 'the greatness of this deed is [yet] too great' (Nietzsche 1974: 181 – para. 125). Observing us, Nietzsche's madman sees that 'this deed is still more distant from them than the most distant stars – *and yet they have done it themselves*' (Nietzsche 1974: 182 – para. 125 – his emphasis). The void is yet to be encompassed and filled, yet to be (fully) known. Connolly provides a compact account of how Nietzsche saw the consequences:

> Once the import of the death of God becomes apparent to those who killed him, the 'will to truth' will appear as the will to impose human form upon the world and then to treat the imposition as if it were a discovery. The more tenacious that will is the more insistent it will have to be in making the world over to fit into its capacities for knowing and the more ruthless it will have to be with those people, actions and events deemed by it to be abnormal, irrational, perverse, unnatural or anomalous. In a world without a divine designer knowing is not a correspondence but an imposition of form upon the objects of knowledge.
>
> (Connolly 1988: 10)

The mythic function of endowing form is entrusted to individual thought which names and orders and which now confers force: 'whatever it touches it immediately causes to move' (Foucault 1970: 327). Hence, 'the one great difference' between modern societies and those based on myth is 'the presence, in the majority of the individuals who constitute modern societies, of a personal

thinking' (Eliade 1968: 24). This thinking individual is constitutively set against the world of myth: again, 'the opposition of
enlightenment to myth is expressed in the opposition of the . . .
individual ego to multifarious fate' (Adorno and Horkheimer
1979: 46). Now, says Legendre, 'we have to do the work of the
Gods' (Legendre 1990: 11). Thought, or, as it is often called in this
context, reason becomes a universal attribute of the individual in
such collective forms as 'man' and humanity. The individual is not,
however, just the transcendent 'nexus of representation and
being' (Foucault 1970: 42). There is more work of the gods, or of
their mediating heroes, to be done. In his wonderful condensation
of the mechanics of myth, in *The Age of Anxiety*, Auden bids us
mourn for the lawgiver 'tall Agrippa who touched the sky'. Even
the gods are bereft for:

> Conjured no more
> By his master music to wed
> Their truths to times, the Eternal Objects
> Drift about in a daze
>
> (Auden 1948: 99)

It is the individual who now mediates between the transcendent
and the real, who now weds truths to times. The displacement of
myth is completed when 'man' comes to be subjected to 'the
sciences of man and society' (Foucault 1970). This subjection,
paradoxically, marks a final liberation, or possibility of liberation,
since the sciences are 'of' man in two senses – they are about 'him'
but they are also 'his'. Thought comes to include 'man's' ability to
conceive of and determine 'his' own being. There is now nothing
ontologically prior to the individual.

I will now begin to orient that modern perspective towards its
mythic character. The perspective, in its own terms, is the dia-
metric opposition of myth. With myth, forms of the real result
from participation in a sacred realm. Knowledge and control of
the real come from locating its origin in the sacred. It is the
unchanging sacred which creates an 'absolute' reality, which
endows it with 'force, effectiveness, and duration' (Eliade 1965: 11,
17). Hence, the 'primitive's obsession with the real, his thirst for
being' (Eliade 1965: 11). This, although in somewhat more elevated terms, is a rendition of the theme of the absolute subjection
of the savage mind to the trammels of superstition and tradition.
Here, I will make another of those occasional forays into what the

ancients and the primitives were like. As we saw earlier, Leach's analysis of myths of virgin birth and Malinowski's account of the Trobriands show that clear distinctions are drawn by 'primitives' between myth and history (Leach 1969: 85ff.; Malinowski 1961: 299, 303). We could add to this Lévi-Strauss's denial of difference between modes of primitive thought and modern, scientific thought (Lévi-Strauss 1968: 230). There are numerous, more tangible indications. The feast of fools, the Saturnalia and other occasions of the temporary reversal of mythic reality, in the erection of contrary myths, make no sense without the reflective perception by the participants that such a reality is limited and not existentially encompassing.

It is the moderns, rather, who are caught within a pervasive mythic reality even if, perhaps, in a way different from that attributed to the primitives and the ancients:

> In the enlightened world, mythology has entered into the profane. In its blank purity, the reality which has been cleansed of demons and their conceptual descendants assumes the numinous character which the ancient world attributed to demons.
>
> (Adorno and Horkheimer 1979: 28)

What results is not, as the claims for Enlightenment would have it, the destruction of myth but, rather, its perfection. The creative force now brought to bear on the world is unitary, inescapable and knows no limits. The profane is swept up into a sacred and panurgic 'man', not as a realm of already fixed resolution but as a project and a progression towards that resolution. For the perfection of beginnings in pre-modern myth is substituted the perfection of ending. There is an integral connection between the specific Western construction of reality as unitary, exclusive and objectively knowable and the construction of the individual as the pre-social, the ultimate and sufficient site of knowing and acting on that reality. The subject is invested with a capacity to know universally, a capacity responsive to universal forms of reality:

> The mind must abandon itself to the abundance of phenomena and gauge itself constantly by them. For it may be sure that it will not get lost, but that instead it will find here its own real truth and standard. Only in this way can the genuine correlation of subject and object, of truth and reality, be achieved.
>
> (Cassirer 1955: 9)

Such confidence is abundantly justified for, in the perfection of myth, subject and reality are matched. To a conscious, purposive subjectivity corresponds an instrumentally ordered reality. The 'unconscious' is given operative existence so far as it corrects pathologies within the conscious in its relation to reality. There are, of course, one or two contradictions entailed in this mythic elevation of the individual, not least how it can persist in an administered world, to borrow Adorno's phrase. I will pursue this in chapter 5.

This elevation, as I indicated earlier, is not yet a triumphant resolution. It is a project and a progression. Not all has yet been subordinated to the manipulative sway of the subject. In modern mythology, the subject is joined with the progression of subordination and with that which remains unsubordinated. These three elements combine in the sacralizing of certain entities, of modern 'Eternal Objects'. The mechanisms of recognition yet denial of myth involved here are delineated in Lefort's account of the 'discourse' of 'bourgeois ideology':

> It is organized in terms of a split between *ideas* and the supposed *real*. The external character of the 'elsewhere', linked to religious or mythical knowledge, is effaced, but the discourse refers back to itself only via the detour of the transcendence of ideas. The text of ideology is written in capital letters, whether it is a question of Humanity, Progress, Nature, Life, or of the key principles of bourgeois democracy inscribed on the pediment of the Republic, or even of Science and Art, but also of Property, Family, Order, Society, Nation.
>
> (Lefort 1986: 205 – his emphasis)

As I will often illustrate, what characterizes this overcrowded pantheon is that its inhabitants combine the three elements I have just mentioned – the subordinating subject, the progression of subordination and what remains unsubordinated. Although my concern is not with the pantheon's exhaustive membership, to it could be added the Subject itself and Law. The thing about 'ruling ideas' is that they rule (cf. Marx and Engels 1974: 64). In mythic terms, these ideas are exemplary, or in Lefort's:

> These ideas are both representations and 'rules', in the sense that they imply a certain way of acting which is consistent with

37

the idea. The ideas thus give rise to an opposition between the subject who speaks and acts in accordance with the rule, and the 'other' who has no access to the rule and is therefore deprived of the status of the subject. The opposition is expressed in a series of dichotomies; worker/bourgeois, savage/civilized, mad/normal, child/adult. Across these dichotomies there emerges a 'natural being', a sub-social, sub-human sphere, the image of which underpins the affirmation of a society above nature. By drawing a distinction between society and that which lies below it, in an underworld of seedy chaos which allegedly threatens the social order, bourgeois ideology seeks to conceal any divisions which exist within society.

(see Thompson 1986: 17)

This ideology serves 'the function of re-establishing the dimension of society "without history" at the very heart of historical society' (Lefort 1986: 201).

'Idea' and its avatars can be seen as myth not very heavily disguised. They provide transcendent origins for 'rules' which are exemplary yet also operatively real in their constitution of identity and the validation of proper conduct. They would seem to body forth a force able to act on and form reality but a force which still leaves the rules set apart from what they affect, leaves them assured and inviolable. Strathern remarks that with 'western society', there is a 'conceptual split between social action which incorporates the ideal, the normative, and what that action controls/regulates/ modifies. Certain types of behaviour thus have the potential for transforming others' (Strathern 1985: 128). The law as it operated on the Haida Indians in Goodrich's story, which I outlined earlier, instances myth in all these terms (Goodrich 1990: chapter 6).

The argument, I hope, is beginning to reveal myth as powerfully operative within modernity but I have yet to reconcile the presence of myth with modernity's specific rejection of a limited, mythic world. Modernity makes an exclusive claim to the unlimited or to the totality. It also involves the invention of 'man', as both the locus of knowledge and 'a source of order for the totality' (Foucault 1970: 313). But man is also an object of that knowledge. 'He' is known through that knowledge, through the human sciences, as a creature of 'finitude and limits': 'we know that man is finite, as we know the anatomy of the brain, the mechanics of production costs, or the system of Indo-European conjugation' (Foucault 1970: 313–14). Man is thus, in Foucault's synopsis, 'a strange empirico-transcendental doublet', able to acquire empirically the contents of knowledge of which 'he' is an object and able to exist transcendentally 'as a pure form immediately present to those contents' (Foucault 1970: 320–1). How is such mythic transcendence achieved and sustained? The answer, as I show in chapter 5, is complex but Foucault provides the beginnings of one:

> This primary discovery of finitude is really an unstable one; nothing allows it to contemplate itself; and would it not be possible to suppose that it also promises that very infinity it refuses, according to the system of actuality? The evolution of the species has perhaps not reached its culmination; forms of production and labour are still being modified, and perhaps one day man will no longer find the principle of his alienation in his labour, or the constant reminder of his limitations in his needs; nor is there any proof that he will not discover symbolic systems sufficiently pure to dissolve the ancient opacity of historical languages. Heralded in positivity, man's finitude is outlined in the paradoxical form of the endless; rather than the rigour of a limitation, it indicates the monotony of a journey which, though it probably has no end, is nevertheless perhaps not without hope.
>
> (Foucault 1970: 314)

As a vicarious agenda for man, this is uncharacteristically if not uniquely subdued. Such depictions of an ontologic destination or direction are usually more roseate and more resolute, providing a charter of progression, even a project, which 'man' in 'making himself' comes increasingly to control or identify with, whether in the projection of an evolutionary progress, a universal spirit, or civilization, to name but a few variants.

The contrast between this and the world of myth is supposedly striking. It can be summarized starkly through Puech's account of time and 'the Greeks':

> Dominated by an ideal of intelligibility which finds authentic and full being only in that which is in itself and remains identical with itself, in the eternal and immutable, the Greeks regarded movement and change as inferior degrees of

reality, in which, at best, identity can be apprehended in the form of permanence and perpetuity, hence of recurrence.

(Puech 1957: 40)

But there is no contrast, I argue, between this and the fantastic realm of the 'Idea' and its avatars which we have just encountered. These entities repeatedly order the world whilst sustaining an immutability and an apartness from it. They are reified and preserved in the operation of abstraction, in 'our craving for generality' (Wittgenstein 1958: 18). Each, within its domain, reduces 'the world as chaotic, manysided and disparate' to 'the known, one, and identical' (see Adorno and Horkheimer 1979: 39).

How can these Eternal Objects be reconciled with charters of progression? There are various mythic strategies for doing this. In one strategy, mythic objects are transposed from an historical dimension of change and contingency to one where meaning is endowed in terms of an elevated universal nature. Barthes saw this shift as definitive of modern myth (Barthes 1973: 142). A comparable autonomy is achieved when the Object takes form as the distinct culmination of a progression, as in certain ideas of 'bourgeois law' where it assumes an apartness and independence from the evolution that produced it (Pashukanis 1978: 71). These two strategies could be seen as aspects of the predominant strategy in modern myth, a strategy, of which the present state of the Object is an interim apotheosis, one which rejects its preceding being but which also contains that being and prefigures all that the Object is yet to become. In this strategy, the story is one of progression, but, in a seemingly subsidiary way, the story assumes an entity that is in progression. The entity is both part of the progression and the progression is in it. Thus, there can be 'scientific' and 'historical' stories of the progress, or the evolution, or the development of Law, of *the* Family and so on.

Although taking identity in a supposed rejection of myth, progression is itself a mythic force, one that I will show later to be central in modern myth. It does figure in modern accounts of myth but the part given to it there is usually subordinated. The myth of origins and of the return of origins is elevated as definitive of myth. Myths of progression – millenarian and redemptive myths, myths of heroic voyage and discovery – are uncomfortably relegated to sub-types (e.g. Eliade 1965). Rendering what is different as a variation of the same is itself a ploy used in myth for dealing with contradiction (see e.g. Leach 1969: 31). A reverse ploy is the transformation of entities and qualities into their opposites. The limited force of progression, by being set in opposition to limited myth, is rendered limitless. It sustains that quality of the limitless by being so constituted in negation and by extending the principle of negation to all of its operation. Any point of progression is simply different to what it was and to what it is to be. The present continually and mythically points beyond itself. With each of its intrinsically mutable moments, it implicates its origins and all that has followed them. The law, for example, is a 'presence which implies the totality of its history, but this implication is not logical or historical; rather, it is traditional and mythic', again to borrow the point from Goodrich and Hachamovitch (1991: 174). Such origins will be less than directly exemplary. They will usually be the abode of savagery. And, as with typical myth, knowledge of origins is needed to control that which so originates – to control our savage passions, for example.

Being constituted in negation, progression is not, in its terms, tied to any specific limiting conditions, to an inexorable fate or to a perennial nature of 'man'. Present inadequacies – the failure of law, an error of science – are but portents of their supersession. Progression, that is, provides an infinitely responsive, mythic mediation between the inviolable Eternal Objects and an operative finitude which would otherwise be seen to impinge on and alter them. The various practical forms of progression, such as progress, development and evolution, are not limiting in this. They are effectively synonyms of progression. In its freedom from limiting conditions, progression becomes a force of universal transformation. It is not tied to any particular place or period. Here is another perfection of myth, of a white mythology in the sense of the mythology of the West. Universal becoming is the prerogative of the West. It is 'enacted in the destiny of sedentary peoples' (Levinas 1979: 46). Non-Western 'others' come to be known and possessed within that universality, the knowledge of which can only be acquired by those others if and to the extent that they can enter positively into this universality. Effectiveness requires an identification with the sacred force of myth: 'He that believeth on me, the works that I do shall he do also' (John 14: 12). Any revelation that there are limits after all in the universality of the West is but the indication of passing imperfection which progression continually transcends. With these closures around progression, 'others' cannot speak or even seek the truth without first shedding their otherness. The very modes and possibilities of escape are contained in a Western progression, in the grandest of 'grand narratives' – the liberation of humanity (see Lyotard 1984: chapter 9).

Narrative becomes inextricably the form of that mythic ordering constructed or discovered in progression. Narrative is not the superseded preserve of 'simpler' peoples. Their myths are often of such labyrinthine complexity as to be irreducible to narrative. No matter what its uses elsewhere, narrative is a simple mode of mastery characteristic of the West. Through narrative, in mythic style, order is created and sustained in tightly linear and irreversible sequences flowing from an origin or an original transition. Through narrative, progressive domination and hierarchy integrally correspond to the sequence's forward thrust. Individual and collective development become heroic and arduous journeys towards an ultimate realization or site of redemption. We can see progression thus pervasively informing Western knowledge through, for example, the dedicated acquisitiveness of Habermas's search for 'the development of normative structures' (Habermas 1979: chapter 4). In that search, a universality increasingly coming to include all persons, who are increasingly coming to be rational and autonomous, is traced in sequential progressions within the biological evolution of 'man', within social evolution, within the development of ego and group identity, within individual and social psychology, and more.

Myth thus ventures forth to create the real, to endow it with 'forms and norms' (Eliade 1965: 10). It provides an exemplary model, a configuration of rules, against which the profane can be evaluated and, if found correspondent, granted presence, reality and validity. As such a guide and measure, myth is an operative reality. No matter what its more attenuated meanings, found in the structure of mind or of a text or anywhere else, myth has an accessible meaning in use and in rituals of use. All of which is not merely a matter of the potentially real being gauged against the perennial fixity in myth. Myth is creative not just in providing an origin but in being a sustained creative force extending itself to and ordering a temporal world, mediating continually between it and the sacred. Thus the lawgiver 'tall Agrippa' who, by wedding the truths of Eternal Objects to times:

Healed the abyss
Of torpid instinct and trifling flux
Laundered it, lighted it, made it lovable with
Cathedrals and theories

(Auden 1948: 98)

It is in this way that myth can be considered poetic, a poetry which, for Vico, is 'not written for aesthetic reasons to delight the mind and adorn a drab world' but poetry as 'a necessity', poetry which imagines forth, 'shaping the several features of the external world into a concrete image' (see Munz 1973: 107). Although this poetry is denied in a world of instrumental reason and the positivist expectation of discovering merely what is, this is nonetheless a necessary, existent poetry. It thus contrasts with mythopoeic calls to reinstate the poetic and the mythic in a world where it is not, with calls to re-enchant that world and to recover what 'time's disasters' have 'utterly consumed' (Leopardi 1966: 233).

Modern myth, although distinct in ways, is nevertheless myth. Its mythic character is ostensibly shed in the elevation of a diachrony which opposes and displaces the timeless and transcendent. Yet we can pull apart the uniform reign of temporality to reveal its dependence on myth. Modern myth, however, in its claims to fullness and totality, cannot admit of a position from which its contours can be traced. They have to be found in what the myth denies or negates. I will now seek out 'the fabulous scene that has produced it' (Derrida 1982: 213).

3

THE MYTHIC FOUNDATION OF MODERN LAW

What sacred games shall we have to invent?
(Nietzsche 1974: 181 – para. 124)

ORIGINS

To continue with borrowed beginnings, this time from Habermas:

> With varying content, the term 'modern' again and again
> expresses the consciousness of an epoch that relates itself to
> the past of antiquity, in order to view itself as the result of a
> transition from the old to the new . . . . The project of mod-
> ernity formulated in the 18th century by the philosophers of
> the Enlightenment consisted in their efforts to develop ob-
> jective science, universal morality and law and autonomous
> art according to their inner logic.
>
> (Habermas 1985: 3, 9)

This was a culmination yet rejection of what had gone before. All
things were made new or at least seen anew. This particular
modernity set itself against the reign of myth: 'Enlightenment
contradicts myth' and 'enlightened thinking has been understood
as an opposition and counterforce to myth' (Habermas 1987: 107).
'The program of Enlightenment was the disenchantment of the
world: the dissolution of myths and the substitution of knowledge
for fancy' (Adorno and Horkheimer 1979: 3). This newly created
world confronted a mythic realm of closed yet multiple meaning,
a realm of the transcendent location of origin and identity. With
Enlightenment the transcendent was brought to earth. 'Man' was
to be the measure of man. There is no need of a mythic mediation
between the real and the transcendental. Meaning was now

44

unified. The transcendental and the limit it imposed on thought and being were the timorous restraints men had placed on themselves in bygone ages. With 'the intoxication of Enlightenment' (see Strakosch 1967: 121), man stood alone daring now to know and, in boundless thought, bringing a unifying reason and knowledge to bear on the dark places. Nothing could remain ultimately intractable or mysterious. Reality and its divisions no longer took identity from their place within an enclosing mythic order – they were manifestations of a process of discovery and realization. When this process reaches the limits of its appropriation of the world, Enlightenment creates the very monsters against which it so assiduously sets itself. These monsters of race and nature mark the outer limits, the intractable 'other' against which Enlightenment pits the vacuity of the universal and in this opposition gives its own project a palpable content. Enlightened being is what the other is not. Modern law is created in this disjunction.

THE HEAVENLY CITY

In debunking the philosophers of Enlightenment, Carl Becker equated the domain to which they would lay claim with the Heavenly City of Augustine:

> In God's appointed time, the Earthly City would come to an end, the earth itself be swallowed up in flames. On that last day good and evil men would be finally separated. For the recalcitrant there was reserved a place of everlasting punishment; but the faithful would be gathered with God in the Heavenly City, there in perfection and felicity to dwell forever.
>
> (Becker 1932: 6)

There are even more venerable precedents and ones more apt 'in the enlightened world [where] mythology has entered into the profane ' (Adorno and Horkheimer 1979: 28) – particularly John's evocation in *Revelation* 21 of 'a new heaven and a new earth'. Once God has made 'all things new':

> the tabernacle of God is with men, and he will dwell with them, and they shall be his people, and God himself shall be with them, and be their God.
>
> (John 21: 3)

45

There follows the ravishing evocation of 'that great city, the holy Jerusalem, descending out of heaven from God'. It is a city infused with the presence of God:

> And I saw no temple therein: for the Lord God Almighty and the Lamb are the temple of it.
> And the city had no need of the sun, neither of the moon, to shine in it: for the glory of God did lighten it, and the Lamb is the light thereof.
> And the nations of them which are saved shall walk in the light of it.
>
> (John 21: 22–4)

The saved are distinguished from those less than committed to an exclusive truth – from 'the fearful, and unbelieving . . . sorcerers, and idolaters, and all liars' and others, all of whom are banished to 'the second death'. These are, of course, themes which have the most profound and extensive resonance throughout the myths of Western Christianity and I will be seeking to show how they imbue Enlightenment and its law.

Returning for now to Becker, he says that his aim is 'to show that the *Philosophes* demolished the Heavenly City of St Augustine only to rebuild it with more up-to-date materials': 'the Heavenly City thus shifted to earthly foundations' (Becker 1932: 31, 49). The terms of the shift are by now well rehearsed: for example, now 'man is capable, guided solely by the light of reason and experience, of perfecting the good life on earth' (Becker 1932: 102). My concern is not immediately with such a claim as this, whether as a supreme good or whether as 'disaster triumphant throughout the earth' (Adorno and Horkheimer 1979: 3). Either view flatters Enlightenment and ultimately accedes to the universality of its reach. My concern with Enlightenment as myth sees it in the terms of the particular and the exotic attributed to those 'others' banished from its truth and being. To focus my enquiry, I will use the image of the Heavenly City but in ways different now to Becker's account.

The mythological city is one form of the powerful symbolism of the centre. The centre – whether a city or temple, a sacred mountain or the Garden of Eden – was a foundation and a source of creation, the point at which the chaos of pre-creation was ordered or crushed, and the point where a transcendentally ordered realm met and conferred a unified, 'enduring, effective' reality on the world (Eliade 1965: 18; see also Goodrich and Hachamovitch 1991: 169–72). The centre was the very image of the world, the *imago mundi*. It pervaded and consecrated all the world's space. But not everything yet partakes of its being:

> For example, desert regions inhabited by monsters, uncultivated lands, unknown seas on which no navigator has dared to venture, do not share with the city of Babylon, or the Egyptian nome, the privilege of a differentiated prototype. They correspond to a mythical model, but of another nature: all these wild, uncultivated regions and the like are assimilated to chaos; they still participate in the undifferentiated, formless modality of pre-Creation.
>
> (Eliade 1965: 9)

In some mythologies a metropolitan creation acts on this modality of pre-creation in an expansionary way:

> Settlement in a new, unknown, uncultivated country is equivalent to an act of Creation. When the Scandinavian colonists took possession of Iceland . . . and began to cultivate it, they regarded this act neither as an original undertaking nor as human and profane work. Their enterprise was for them only the repetition of a primordial act: the transformation of chaos into cosmos by the divine act of Creation. By cultivating the desert soil, they in fact repeated the act of the gods, who organized chaos by giving it forms and norms. Better still, a territorial conquest does not become real until after – more precisely, through – the ritual of taking possession, which is only a copy of the primordial act of the Creation of the World. In Vedic India the erection of an altar dedicated to Agni constituted legal taking possession of a territory.
>
> (Eliade 1965: 10–11)

Similarly, 'the English navigators took possession of conquered countries in the name of the king of England, new Cosmocrator' (Eliade 1965: 11).

The dimensions and dynamic of the Earthly City of Enlightenment seem at first to be markedly similar to the celestial. Its claim to unify and order reality is no less encompassing. And there also remain strange regions beyond the elect community of enlightened nations, as they were called – regions to be continually discovered and reduced to order. Such a ready resemblance surely cannot withstand the necessary history of difference between the enlightened and the pre-modern world. But such a foundational difference, I now argue, incorporates the very dimension of myth that it would seek to deny.

What Enlightenment and modernity supposedly reject, in a word, is transcendence. The key divide posited by Eliade is one between a mythic world where 'neither the objects of the external world nor human acts . . . have an autonomous intrinsic value' and a modern world where they do (Eliade 1965: 3). Mythically, 'objects or acts acquire value, and in so doing become real, because they participate, after one fashion or another, in a reality that transcends them' (Eliade 1965: 3–4). Such things once 'shone differently because a god shone through them' (Nietzsche 1974: 196 – para. 152). In the uniform light of modernity, there is no room for a duality of meaning or for any ultimate ambiguity. What we have instead is the elevation of 'the objects' in a sense encompassing not just a separate material thing but also a distinct constellation of action, such as law. Objects have and maintain identity 'in themselves, complete, self-referring and proper' (Douzinas and Warrington 1991: 10).

I will begin to extract the mythic dimensions of the object in terms of its origin, its function and its relation to other objects. Enlightenment's obsession with origins is perhaps the most obvious substitute for the mythically transcendent. The object could no longer take its being from the transcendent source provided in a myth of origin. Its essence now was simply found in its origin. Origin revealed the object in its pristine simplicity. Thus Cassirer, in remarking on the 'complete diversity, this heterogeneity and fluidity' of psychology in the eighteenth century, finds that 'closer inspection reveals the solid grounds and the permanent elements underlying the almost unlimited mutability of psychological phenomena': 'if we trace psychological forms to their sources and origins, we always find such unity and relative simplicity' (Cassirer 1955: 16–17). Originary time is connected with the present object in a process of development or civilization in which the continuity of the object is sustained even while it changes. This process was recounted, as we shall see later, in fantastic stories devised in the names of reason and history. Of the infinity of possible objects, narratives were told of some only, and these were told with the constant repetition that characterizes the operation of myth. They included tales of society, law, property and other Eternal Objects such as I described in the last chapter. Eternal Objects dramatically instance the mythic function of the object. Objects provide 'exemplary models' against which the validity or reality of an act is measured (Eliade 1965: 28). Objects, to borrow Lefort's terms again, are 'both representations and "rules", in the sense that they imply a certain way of acting which is consistent with' the object (see Thompson 1986: 17). And those who act in ways consistent with Eternal Objects are included in the ranks of the elect – a point I will develop shortly. So much for the origin and function of objects. I will now look at their mythic dimension in the relationship between them.

Despite their erection in denial of a mythic order or a mythic lawgiver, objects in modernity do not 'drift about in a daze' (Auden 1948: 99). The universalist thrust of Enlightenment places the object in an integral relation to the 'general' conceived in such terms as universal ordering and reason. What was general had the potential of being known completely, even if some saw that as incapable of final realization. But the shortfall was no restraint on a totalizing ambition. There were to be no ultimate limits. Multiplicity and difference could be safely sought in the steady anticipation that they would return to an assured unity:

> The path of thought then, in physics as in psychology and politics, leads from the particular to the general; but not even this progression would be possible unless every particular as such were already subordinated to a universal rule, unless from the first the general were contained, so to speak embodied, in the particular.
>
> (Cassirer 1955: 20)

This dynamic of identity was taken even further:

> One should not seek order, law, and 'reason' as a rule that may be grasped and expressed prior to the phenomena, as their *a priori*; one should rather discover such regularity in the phenomena themselves, as the form of their immanent connection.
>
> (Cassirer 1955: 9)

This alternation between the general and the particular cannot, in modernity, be accommodated in distinct realms as they would so readily be in other mythologies. What unites them and sustains the unity of being, apart from the formulaic gymnastics of the type just instanced, are Eternal Objects. These, in mythic style, mediate between the general and the specifically particular by appropriating the quality of the universal to themselves. Occidental forms, as Eternal Objects, thus provide exemplary models of what the world really is or should be. Let us take property as an instance. As an 'external', reified object, it is suffused with the palpable and the specific. Yet it is also elevated in terms no less extensive than those attributed to the transcendence of myth. It is, to summarize various formulations of Enlightenment, the foundation of civilization, the very motor-force of the origin and development of society, the provocation to self-consciousness and the modality of appropriating nature: 'Property is man', if 'only civilized man': it is identified with 'individuality, liberty and history' and is 'as precious as life itself': it is thus readily seen in terms of the 'sacred' and the 'eternal' (see Kelley 1984a: 129–33). What is being universalized here is a particular form of Occidental property. Where it is absent there can only be its precursors or savagery.

There are general elements combined within the Eternal Object. These, as I peremptorily indicated in the last chapter, comprise the subordinating subject, the progression of subordination and that which remains unsubordinated. I will say something more about these, particularly the third. Both the subject and progression were dealt with extensively in the last chapter and I will return to them in the next; the third I consider here in its form of nature. I will look at the subject and progression mainly as a prelude to the account of nature. Through the subject, whether singularly as the individual or collectively as humanity, any action or object can be integrated with the most pervasive and extensive reality. There is an impetus towards creation enabling this to be done which emanates from a particular facility of thought, reason or the mind. 'The highest energy and deepest truth of the mind do not consist in going out into the infinite, but in the mind's maintaining itself against the infinite and proving in its pure unity equal to the infinity of being' (Cassirer 1955: 38).

It is progression which comprehensively enfolds the transcendent within the temporal. Mundane reality is sustained in the prospect of 'perfectibility' – one of 'the words without which no enlightened person could reach a restful conclusion' (Becker 1932: 47). Even the professedly anti-Utopian succumbed to its necessity. So, for Bentham, the radiant potential of his principle of utility was such that:

> though no one now living may be permitted to enter into this land of promise, yet he who shall contemplate it in its vastness and beauty may rejoice, as did Moses, when on the verge of the desert, from the mountain top, he saw the length and breadth of that good land into which he was not permitted to enter and take possession.
>
> (see Holdsworth 1952: 79)

It is, in sum, difficult not to see the discovery of progress in the eighteenth century as myth triumphant. Although the closest mythic analogue may be with myths of the heroic search or voyage, or even the myths of eschatology, progress also evokes origins. Progress does not just go somewhere, it comes from somewhere. Progression is the continuity of an origin, of the passage from pre-creation to the manifest. The lineary progression of the West is one of constant and accumulative creation. This is, nonetheless, an ordered, even restrained creation. Progress would always be potentially disruptive unless it were reduced to an orderly course in nature. Eventually, progress comes to be seen not merely as a matter of expectation or aspiration, but as itself one of nature's laws – that story is taken up in the next chapter.

NATURE AND THE DEIFICATION OF LAW

'Order is Heav'n's first law' (Pope 1950: 132 – Epistle IV, line 49). When the Heavenly City is brought to Earth, order becomes the first law of nature. Before then, the accepted histories have it, God was considered the supreme lawgiver. Law had to conform ultimately to this mythic origin for its being or validity. No matter how ingenious the scholastic solutions applying God's word to the mundane world, and no matter how mysterious 'his' ways, God remained the necessary and unavoidable source of law's being. Enlightenment replaces God with nature. In terms of the origin myths of modern science, the deific obstacle to humanity's progress in knowledge is eliminated, constraining superstition gives way to incandescent truth, man unaided at last dares to know, and so on. Thus:

> all we have to to is put aside the hindrances which heretofore have delayed the progress of natural science and prevented it from resolutely pursuing its path to the end. What always prevented the human mind from achieving a real conquest

51

of nature and from feeling quite at home there was the unfortunate tendency to ask for a realm beyond. If we set aside this question of transcendence, nature ceases at once to be a mystery. Nature is not mysterious and unknowable, but the human mind has enveloped it in artificial darkness . . . . The riddle of nature vanishes for the mind which dares to stand its ground and cope with it. For such a mind finds no contradictions and partitions but only one being and one form of law.

(Cassirer 1955: 65)

This revolution, so the story continues, is accompanied by a basic change in the nature of law. To adopt Althusser's way of putting it, law previously had been solely a matter of '*commandment*. It thus needed a will to order and wills to obey . . . . Law having only one structure, divine law, natural law and positive (human) laws could be discussed *in the same sense* . . . . Divine law dominated all law' (Althusser 1972: 31–2 – his emphasis). But this is changed and nature has laws which are not orders but simply order – a new and 'inexorable regularity and legality' (Hodgen 1964: 450). But, I will argue, the mythic dimension attributed to the prior order of God also characterizes the new order of nature. What happens is that God becomes captured by 'his' creation. Malebranche was a deft exponent of the process:

The will of God is only the love He directs toward His own attributes . . . . Therefore He can only will and act according to that which He is, only in a manner which bears the character of His attributes. [This is] because He is glorified by being what He is, and by possessing the perfections included in His essence. In a word, [it is] because he cannot contradict Himself, cannot will against the eternal and immutable perfections of his essence.

(see Walton 1972: 38)

'Order is . . . [the] inviolable Law' of God's action (Walton 1972: 38). The presence of order and uniformity in nature's laws still required, for Newton and others, a divine lawgiver. After chastising Christ for attributing a particular will or design to God the Father – for saying that the Father would be concerned 'to clothe the lilies of the field and to preserve the least hair of his disciples' head' – Malebranche asserts that 'order does not permit that [God] have practical *volontés* proper to the execution of his design . . . . He must not disturb the simplicity of his ways' (Riley 1986: 35, 40). God is thus confined to a general will, to acting 'as a consequence of general laws which he has established' (see Riley 1986: 29). God is hardly now in a position to resist expulsion from nature altogether – a kind of reverse Eden. What is perhaps worse, there were great ancestor figures of modern law, such as Grotius, who still attributed the new law ultimately to God but nonetheless recognized that God was not strictly necessary for nature. If God persists, 'he' no longer possesses nature but is possessed by it. It is now a matter of 'the laws of nature and of nature's God', as the US Declaration of Independence has it.

This outcome at first seems contrary to the place that nature usually finds in myth. Nature and culture are there placed in opposition. Culture advances by taming and appropriating nature. But the laws of nature and of nature's God inhabit the world, including its culture, as pervasively and comprehensively and in as unifying a way as did the pre-modern deity – 'the law that preserved the stars from wrong was also the rule of duty' (Willey 1940: 14).

For Grotius, as the modern begetter of law for an entire world, the impulse towards sociality provided by 'human nature . . . is the mother of natural law' (see Robinson *et al.* 1985: 359). To establish this natural law, he looked to writers of antiquity as well as to more contemporary religious and juristic sources, all of them understandably Occidental. In all: 'that is according to the law of nature which is believed to be such among all nations or among all those that are more advanced in civilization' (see Stein 1980: 4). The natural law of Enlightenment remained within the tradition of Grotius with somewhat more emphasis on 'scientific' modes of reason and calculation. Reason, in turn, was seen as typical of 'man'. It was both part of man's nature and an imperative guide to what that nature was. All versions of Enlightenment natural law shared the same universal scale and the same partaking in an objective nature.

This story of law's domestication of the deity is a comparatively short one because, in terms of another story, objective natural law did not endure as a basis for practical legal regulation. Elements of it seem to persist in law, as we shall see, but objective natural law endures more fully as scientific administration. That particular story is taken up in later chapters. There is now division in a once unitary law, a division between 'the law that preserved the stars from wrong' and 'the rule of duty'. That rule is located in the tradition of law as command, a tradition which persisted and was not wholly subordinated in objective order.

Accounts of law as the acts of a sovereign will are every bit as ancient as the equation of law with a set order. The division between the two types of law is tied up with competing Occidental deities. One is the origin and ruler of the cosmos and can alter it at will. Although this god's ways remain ultimately mysterious, they do have to be known if they are to be mythically operative. The primary form of this knowledge is revelation. The other deity is that captured by 'his' own creation. This god is allowed to act only in accordance with the divine order. The primary mode of acquiring knowledge in this scheme is reason. Both of these gods continue to inhabit law but the predominant story of modern law, one told now in the perspective of the nation-state, attributes precedence to the god of will and revelation. The story is so well known as not to bear repetition without tedium. To summarize, it is a story of the separation and dominance of a secular power in the initial form of the centralizing monarchies of medieval and early modern Europe. Although some god is invoked for a time as a final source of law, political rule assumes a secular sweep in which the divine becomes incidental or irrelevant. Hobbes's Leviathan, that 'mortal god', is a resonant marker of the change (Hobbes 1952: 100). Natural and divine law become subordinate to the self-sufficient determination of positive law – the law posited by the will of the sovereign.

God's surreptitious triumph can, nonetheless, be glimpsed in the composition of modern law. Merely to present modern law's deific attributes could be to parade the obvious. These attributes could appear to be simply the case, just as a mythology should appear. I will attempt to dramatize the argument by resort to Kafka's 'The Great Wall of China': there can be 'no contemporary law' where 'long-dead emperors are set on the throne in our villages, and one that only lives in song recently had a proclamation of his read out by the priest before the altar' (Kafka 1961: 78, 80). We could reduce this in socio-legal terms to a point about limits to law's efficacy but I take it as a point about the mythic being of Occidental law. It cannot be 'contemporary law' drawing together diversities in time and abstracting from it without transcendentally opposing a palpable world that denies transcendence. God similarly persisted in the face of the denials of a profane or profaned world. The god of the Hebrews and the Christians was a jealous god, one who would never relax the totality and the inexorability of 'his' claims to obedience. There could be 'none other gods before me' (Deuteronomy 5: 7). God was the creator of all, sole and omnipotent, pervasive and eternal. Only those who act in accord with the mythic exemplar of God's will or God's law can be saved. Whether or not so to act is a matter for God's subjects in the exercise of that freedom and responsibility which they share with the deity.

Law once bore the characters of God. It explicitly took mythic origins in the godhead. This connection becomes attenuated or, to adopt Derrida's terms, the mythology becomes anaemic or whitened (Derrida 1982: 213). The sovereign is no longer God's earthly representative and is now the autonomous and self-sufficient source of law. Law, once it was processed by Kant, is no longer tied to any extraneous order, now deriving its force and origin purely from its intrinsic being. Yet, despite all this, law does not or cannot assume merely terrestrial dimensions. It continues to bear the characters of God. But it does this now in a mundane world.

We can again attempt to penetrate that world in the drama of difference. When delineating Eternal Objects, I used Strathern's location within 'Western liberal society' of a type of 'social action which incorporates the ideal, the normative' and remains apart from and unaffected by 'what that action controls/regulates/modifies' (Strathern 1985: 128). She arrives at this perception through its difference to the modes of regulation among the people of Hagen in the New Guinea Highlands. With these people, one mode of regulation, such as fighting or gift exchange or 'talk', is deeply influenced by and even transformable into another. Western law, in contrast, is invested with inviolability and transcendence. These qualities are usually put in terms of law's being normative or formal, general or abstract. In practical terms, this entails law's not being able to 'bear very much reality' (cf. Eliot 1935: 49). Law has to be kept at a remove 'from the everyday commitments and discourses of social and political practice and conflict' (Goodrich 1987: 5). For this, it assumes the trappings that keep myth apart from the profane yet make it operative, such as priests/guardians of the myth and its constrained application in ritual. Law's effects are formed magically – that is through 'a method of supporting endeavour to control the environment and social relationships by means where the connection of effort with achievement cannot be measured' (Gluckman 1968: 111). Law, like the deity, creates its own world and the legal reality is the magical effect of invoking formulas within law which are mythically adhered to by priests and people (Hagerström 1953). As magical and transcendent, law cannot be brought into an evaluative, much less definitive comparison with mundane reality.

Law takes on and retains its quality of transcendent effectiveness as an enduring type of sovereign rule. Like the monotheistic sovereign, law is a transcendent unity: the 'inevitability of legal unity is seen as central to the very idea of legal order' (Carty 1991: 182). So, Holdsworth finds, in one of the better stretches of Blackstone's verse, the informing ideal of his great consolidation of English law:

> Observe how parts with parts unite
> In one harmonious rule of right;
> See countless wheels distinctly tend
> By various laws to one great end.

(see Holdsworth 1952: 704)

This harmony and this end come from within law itself. Like its divine counterpart, law is autonomous and self-sustaining. It is independent of any exterior reality. It is not bound by any temporal order: or, more exactly, law's time exists beyond mundane temporality (Goodrich and Hachamovitch 1991: 167, 174). Any past, any future can be integrated into its eternal presence. Space is also transcended. Law has, as Carty puts it, the quality of 'everywhereness' (Carty 1991: 196). 'There cannot be an "absence of law"' (Stone 1964: 24). Law is, in all, possessed of a universality which 'exceeds all finitudes' (Carty 1990: 6). This is a universality which rejects or incorporates the particular. The evanescent particularities of mundane reality are taken up into law and there rendered effective and persistent. 'Reality [is] being adjusted' continually. to a law 'which transforms the social realm so as to render it assimilable to the normative complex' (Lenoble and Ost 1980: 110). Accounts of modern law diverge in the range and force they accord to law's acting on mundane reality. Claims have been made, often in the traditions of objective natural law, for the encompassing ability of law to make or re-make society totally. Such an aspiration was not remote from the makers of the 'liberal' French Code Civil (see Kelley 1984a: 42–5). Bentham, conceiving himself as the Newton of the moral world, combined law's completeness with its limitless sovereignty in the prospect of an eventual attainment of total and 'certain order' (Lieberman 1989: 281). The less ambitious liberal manifestation of law's omnipotence attributes to law not the ability to do everything but the ability to do anything. Law remains pervasive, able to intervene at any point but not intervening at every point. Some areas are supposed to remain characteristically apart, notably a 'private' domain of the subject.

Even in this provisionally limited, liberal mode, law maintains its imperial and universal character against the particular. Law's range of determination remains infinite. As an operative condensation of Enlightenment thought, law becomes:

> an immanent principle that unites the parts into a whole, that makes this whole the object of a general knowledge and will whose sanctions are merely derivative of a judgement and an application directed at the rebellious parts.
>
> (Deleuze and Guattari 1983: 212)

Anything can be made the object of this judgement and application. Along with the generality of its sanctioning force, law demands 'that all sectors of society abandon their autonomy of legal interpretation (that is, of the extent of their obligation) in favour of a single . . . interpretative authority' (Carty 1991: 182). Thus we have replicated in law the 'Christian axiom that custom, history, tradition, were to be conquered in their effectiveness by the word – and the law . . . is little more than the word; "in principio erat verbum"; in the beginning was the word' (Ullmann 1975: 49). What is more, modern law could re-shape the conquered, could 'release norm-contents from the dogmatism of mere tradition and . . . determine them intentionally' (Habermas 1976: 86). So, law's power of positive and universal determination turns, as it were, against social relations to which law was once integrally tied. Law constitutes and empowers the realm of so-called civil privatism which replaces the myriad 'public' realms of pre-modern regulation. This civil privatism came to be permeated by detailed controls of administration and these were ultimately supported by law's dealing with 'the rebellious parts'. The legal subject emerges out of this paradoxical privatism not only as the abstract bearer of legal rights and duties, but also, as we will see in the next chapter, as the possessor of a specific Occidental identity not unlike that possessed by the subject of the Christian god.

We have already encountered another Christian god besides the ineffable, commanding sovereign, and lineaments of this god are also to be found in modern law. With objective natural law, God came to be contained in 'his' creation as 'against the derivation of law from a completely irrational divine will which is impenetrable to human reason' and 'is in the last analysis rooted in divine omnipotence . . . absolutely unconditional and subject to no limiting rules and norms' (Cassirer 1955: 238). This was an old divide, one which had persisted throughout the Middle Ages, to take it no further back. In its modern guise, it is seen in the division between a stable, independent legal order and an earthly form of absolute rule, the commanding sovereign of the Leviathan state (Cassirer 1955: 238). The stable and independent 'rule of law' came to be secured in two ways. In one, legal restraint on the state and some enduring stability of law were set in constitutional provisions or procedures the alteration of which was beyond the normal competence of the state. These were usually based in claims to 'natural' or 'human' rights. In the other mode, restraint was built into the law itself. Most notably, the general will which Malebranche had foisted onto God, in opposition to claims that God could 'command' anything, was an antecedent of the generality that mythically inhabits modern law (Riley 1986). For Rousseau, 'the object of laws is always general'; 'no function which has a particular object belongs to the legislative power', and 'what the sovereign commands with regard to a particular matter' is not 'law but is a decree, an act, not of sovereignty, but of magistracy' (Rousseau 1986: 211–12).

Perhaps the most significant legacy of the god of order is the mythic equation of Occidental law with order. Just as order is Heaven's first law, so 'the law is an order, and therefore all legal problems must be set and solved as order problems' (Kelsen 1967: 192). Through 'legal mytho-logic' there is a 'handling of contradictions in society according to the prescriptions of order' (Lenoble and Ost 1980: 229). But the order secured in law cannot itself now be secured in the order of God or nature. There are limits, as Rousseau observed, to an order achieved in 'the nature of things':

> All justice comes from God, who is its sole source; but if we
> knew how to receive so high an inspiration, we should need

neither government nor laws. Doubtless, there is a universal justice emanating from reason alone; but this justice, to be admitted among us, must be mutual. Humanly speaking, in default of natural sanctions, the laws of justice are ineffective among men . . . . Convention and laws are therefore needed to join rights to duties and refer justice to its object.

(Rousseau 1986: 210)

The willed sanction is thus necessary for modern law. There remains, in all, a persistent contradiction between law as avatar of the god of order and law as avatar of the god of illimitable sovereignty.

The serenity of law as transcendent is further disturbed by a certain popular dimension of law. Ullmann describes 'two contrasting themes which portray the creation of law' in 'the Western world':

Historically speaking, the one called the ascending theme of government and law, can claim priority and appears to be germane alike to lowly and highly developed societies. Its main point is that law-creative power is located in the people itself . . . : the populace at large is considered to be the bearer of the power that creates law either in a popular assembly or diet, or, more usually, in a council or other organ which contains the representatives chosen by the people . . . . Opposed to this ascending theme is the descending one according to which original power is located not in the broad base of the people, but in an otherworldly being, in divinity itself which is held to be the source of all power, public and private. The totality of original power being located in one supreme being was distributed downward – or 'descended from above' – so that the mental picture of a pyramid emerges: at its apex there was the Ruler who had received power from divinity and who distributed it downwards, so that whatever power was found at the base of the pyramid was eventually traceable to the supreme head. But, and this is one of the crucial differences from the ascending theme, the office holders are not representatives: they are only delegates of the supreme Ruler.

(Ullmann 1975: 30–1)

There was a sharp conflict, as Ullmann shows, between these themes in the Middle Ages. The standard account in the modern

59

history of the West is that, with the decline of absolutist sovereignty and the growth of representative government, the ascending theme progressively wins out. Yet predominant jurisprudential accounts persistently and readily see modern law in terms of the descending theme.

We can refine this contrast by following a seeming by-way in histories of Western law, that of custom, as a popular legal form. Other popular dimensions of law will be considered later in this chapter. Through custom, says Ullmann: 'the stark contrast between the descending and ascending theme of government is . . . nakedly revealed' (Ullmann 1975: 63). Even where it was not mediated through a popular assembly, custom in the medieval period was often accorded an efficacy equal to or greater than that of legislation. It was even more frequently esteemed above 'written laws' and could be foundational of these laws. Although custom was based on usage or long acceptance, it was, according to Aquinas, capable of changing in ways 'just as motivated by the reasoned will as are the written changes of statutory law' (Morrall 1980: 75). It could extend beyond the local community. The common law, for example, took some of its origins from general customs of the realm.

Out of the Enlightenment obsession with custom, a different and degraded form emerges. Custom becomes reduced to a peripheral category set in opposition to law through its association with the savage and with those small-scale remnants of a recalcitrant past yet to be transformed in modernity. It is produced by implacable habit and is everything that the reasoned will is not. It is, said Bentham, 'for brutes' – 'written law [being] the law for civilized nations' (Bentham 1970a: 153). Austin followed suit. For him, law as a positive product of the will contrasted essentially with rules that rest on 'brute custom' rather than on 'manly reason' and were thus 'monstrous or crude productions of childish and imbecile intellect' (Austin 1861–3: 58 – I).

The treatment of custom in the English domestic scene had for some purposes to be more tender. The common law was once equated with general customs that were to prevail through 'the whole kingdom' (Blackstone 1825: 66–7 – I). But Blackstone reduced custom to the domination of law and to insignificance. General custom is subjected to the pronouncements of judges, 'the living oracles' of the law, whose judgement and proceedings are 'carefully registered and preserved, under the name of *records*' and whose determinations become a certain and 'permanent rule' (Blackstone 1825: 68 – I – his emphasis). Through this process, the common law, like the legislative sovereign, becomes a transcendent entity – 'a brooding omnipresence in the sky' (Holmes in *Southern Pacific Co. v. Jensen* (1917 244 US 205 at 222)). It becomes positive or posited law, operating and elaborated in officially contained systems which are incompatible with custom, although some patina of its presence, even some custom-like modalities, survive (Simpson 1987: 361).

There still remained a type of custom that was not general but 'particular'. Blackstone adroitly marginalized it: 'for reasons that have been now long forgotten, particular counties, cities, towns, manors and lordships, were very early indulged with the privilege of abiding by their own customs, in contra-distinction to the rest of the nation at large' (Blackstone 1825: 74 – I). Such customs could (and can) only be accorded legal recognition if they surmount a long line of hurdles. To take an example, the mythic grandeur which once attended custom's origin in a 'time whereof the memory of man runneth not to the contrary' is now reduced to a paltry exactitude: 'so that if anyone can show the beginning of it, it is no good custom' (Blackstone 1825: 67,76 – I).

To trespass on the dynamics of another age, and of the next chapter, custom in a broad dimension and the ascending theme can be seen as persisting. In that broad dimension, custom effected and symbolized the unity of the pre-modern community and was its 'common conscience' (Berman 1983: 77). Towards the end of the period of Enlightenment, and in professed reaction against it, Savigny revived a tradition that has since endured in social conceptions of modern law. He discovered that it was not a sovereign will but custom as the 'common consciousness of the people' that was the foundation of law (Savigny 1831: 28, 30). Although the popular dimension of law thus conflicts with law's claim to transcendence, it is subordinated to law as sovereign. Legislation has for Savigny a distinct and necessary existence (Savigny 1831: 104–5). Since it is allowed no specifically determining effect of its own, custom exists in the realm of the vaguely influential, of what ideally should be taken into account in legislating. As with the common law, Savigny's famed idea of law as *Volksgeist*, as the spirit of the people, appropriates custom to a sovereign system leaving only a seductive trace of its presence. The ascending theme, of law in the instance of custom is not accommodated within law but subordinated to its descending theme, leaving the tension between the two unresolved in law.

Drawing back from this account of the deification of law, we are left with a mystery, or with a series of mysteries. Like the god of *Revelation*, myth enters into the great city of the Enlightened world. It disappears within an encompassing and unitary reality. Law cannot now resort to a transcendent source for its origin and identity. God no longer shines through law. Yet the characters of God are preserved within law itself. How, then, can law maintain its transcendent being within a uniform reality, sustaining deific qualities of autonomy, omnipotence, pervasiveness, and so on? Even in its transcendent dimension, law is not coherent for it is imbued with the conflicting gods of Europe, the god of illimitable sovereign will and the god of order who is captured by 'his' own creation. Transcendent law is contradicted as well in law's popular dimension. Law's deific qualities and law's unity and coherence cannot, then, be found in what law is. But law's deific qualities do not allow it to be subordinate in its being to a source outside of itself.

Where or how else can law find that which gives it being, a new 'fabulous scene that has produced it' (Derrida 1982: 213)? It is now found not in terms of what law is but in terms of what law is not. It is found no longer in terms of what law is subordinate to but in terms of what is subordinate to it. Foucault locates at the outset of the modern period a shift in the fundamental mode whereby knowledge is acquired:

> The activity of the mind . . . will . . . no longer consist in *drawing things together*, in setting out on a quest for everything that might reveal some sort of kinship, attraction or secretly shared nature within them, but, on the contrary, in *discriminating*, that is, in establishing their identities . . . . In this sense, discrimination imposes upon comparison the primary and fundamental investigation of difference.
>
> (Foucault 1970: 55 – his emphasis)

Such a mode of difference is not simply abstract or analytical. It has clear contents to do with identity and order. Nor is it simply the discovery of identity and order but their mythic creation through assured thought or reason brought to bear on the world in the project of Enlightenment. When the limits of that creation are met, Enlightenment confronts 'wild uncultivated regions' and an 'undifferentiated . . . pre-creation' (Eliade 1965: 9). This it sets beyond itself, beyond its exemplary models, as its opposition and difference. But this is also its own pre-creation, and Enlightenment finds there its mythic origins. In the taking of identity from these origins, they become something to be departed from and negated rather than something to be positively emulated. They form negative exemplars. Hence, modern myth is the ascent from savagery instead of the descent from gods (cf. Sahlins 1976: 52–3).

In the transforming thought of Enlightenment, culture confronts nature in standard mythic terms. Savages are of nature rather than culture and they are denied transforming thought or reason. Like the devils of Christian belief, to whom they were constantly compared, savages cannot escape the light but are forever cast out by it. The identities of the European and of European law are achieved in their foundational difference from these beings. I will develop that line of argument in the rest of this chapter.

NATURE, RACE AND LAW

Enlightenment inherits and refines a profound division in 'nature' – another obsession of the age. In the Christian tradition, the Pauline 'natural man' has to become a 'new creature' in order to be saved (I Corinthians 2: 14; II Corinthians 5: 17). The old Adam of fallen nature had to be cast out in baptism. In the Thomist rendition, nature is the creation of God; the participation by rational beings in God's rule of his creation takes the form of natural law. The Enlightenment variation is summarized by Jordanova:

> While it is important to realize that nature was endowed with a remarkable range of meanings during the period of the Enlightenment . . . there was also one common theme. Nature was taken to be that realm on which mankind acts, not just to intervene in or manipulate directly, but also to understand and render it intelligible. This perception of nature includes people and the societies they construct. Such an interpretation of nature led to two distinct positions: nature could be taken to be that part of the world which human beings have understood, mastered and made their own. Here, through the unravelling of laws of motion for

63

example, the inner recesses of nature were revealed to the human mind. But secondly, nature was also that which has not yet been penetrated (either literally or metaphorically), the wilderness and deserts, unmediated and dangerous nature.

(Jordanova 1980: 66)

The second position extended to wild and savage people as well as places. It was an old position, one seemingly indistinguishable from the evocation of those wild, uncultivated regions on which creation operates in myth. Similarly, the appropriated nature of the first position seems to correspond to the achieved and differentiated creation of myth. The difference between Enlightenment and mythic conceptions of nature, however, would supposedly lie in the assertion of a unitary reality as opposed to myth's dual dimensions. Appropriated nature cannot be a transcendent prototype and wild nature cannot be a qualitatively different realm of sempiternal monsters and impassable deserts. But these two dimensions of myth can be readily located in Enlightenment once it is appreciated that the division between appropriated and wild nature is itself encompassed by order, leaving an intractable disorder beyond it. The appropriated and the yet-to-be appropriated share in the same universal order of things (see Foucault 1970: 56–7).

It is the sovereign subject who effects a unifying order in nature and who brings things together in order: 'Man's likeness to God consists in sovereignty over existence, in the countenance of the lord and master, and in command' (Adorno and Horkheimer 1979: 9). In terms closer to the times, Enlightenment:

attributes to thought not merely an imitative function but the power and the task of shaping life itself. Thought consists not only in analysing and dissecting, but in actually bringing about that order of things which it conceives as necessary, so that by this act of fulfilment it may demonstrate its own reality and truth.

(Cassirer 1955: viii)

The sovereign subject becomes the illimitable conduit for illimitable thought and reason. Yet the subject also sustains a distinct identity, 'maintaining itself against the infinite' (cf. Cassirer 1955: 38). It is self-sufficient, set apart from and dominant over nature.

This is a primal, sovereign and assured position which recognizes, names and orders from afar. As Linnaeus announces, 'the exact Names of things finally rule' (see Foucault 1970: 159). Human identity, in short, 'contained the nexus of representation and being' (Foucault 1970: 311). Such an identity could not appear in terms of a positive finitude because it could not be any (limited) thing at all. The sovereign subject took identity in difference – its difference from a wild, disordered nature and from, in particular, that 'untamed . . . natural man' wherein, says Hegel of 'the Negro, . . . there is nothing harmonious with humanity' (see Poliakov 1974: 241). In mythic terms, this identity of the sovereign subject comes from the creation of European racism.

Myth's basic function, in its European conception, is the conferring of identity on a people. With the creation of modern European identity in Enlightenment the world was reduced to European terms and those terms were equated with universality. That which stood outside of the absolutely universal could only be absolutely different to it. It could only be an aberration or something other than what it should be. It is thus negatively and inextricably connected to the universal. 'The compass opened . . . the universe' (Montesquieu 1949: 366), and there were no longer multiple worlds and difference could not find refuge from an exclusive universality. 'Now,' as Burke announces, 'the Great Map of Mankind is unrolld at once' (see Marshall and Williams 1982: introductory quotation).

The imperatives of difference had palpable dimensions. 'The eighteenth century proved the golden age of slaving' (Wolf 1982: 196). There was an expansion of colonization and colonial rule became more explicit and comprehensive in its subordination. By 1800 the West already controlled over a third of the earth's surface. With its expansive claim to exclusive rationality, with its arrogation of a universal and uniform knowledge of the world, and with its affirmation of universal freedom and equality, the Enlightenment sets a fateful dimension. Being of humanity and being unfree were incompatible (Rousseau 1986: 186). The all-too-obvious contradiction between Enlightenment thought and practice is mythically resolved by the invention of racism. The Enlightenment gives currency to 'race' in its modern connotation of divisions between people founded on certain physical attributes, usually skin colour. It also affixes to the idea of race three monumental correlates that go to make up racism as it is now called. For racism, differences based on race are fundamental, intractable and unerringly indicative of superiority and inferiority. Those excluded from the domain of knowing, reason, equality and freedom by a buoyant British and French slavery or an expanding colonization are rendered in racist terms as qualitatively different. This was not simply a matter of excluding the enslaved from the realms of liberty and universal law, as Grotius and Locke did (see Davis 1966: 114–15; Locke 1965: 325–6, 366 – paras. 23–4, 85). In the ubiquitous, all-defining gaze of Enlightenment, the enslaved were purposively constructed as essentially different and strange. Through taking identity in opposition to this creation, Europeans become bound in their own being by the terms in which they oppress others (cf. Hegel 1977: 111–19 – B.IV A).

I will take Long's *History of Jamaica* (1774) as a typical account of that essential difference which provided the counter in the making of modern European identity. Given Long's supposedly extreme views, this may seem a tendentious choice. However, Long's racism 'fitted all too well into the pattern of racial and cultural pride already prevalent in English thought' (Curtin 1964: 44). He was indeed to prove the progenitor of scientific racism. The *philosophes*, it could be objected, were more refined and their racism was merely incidental in their work or even humorously intended (see Barker 1981: chapter 4; Davis 1966: 403 – cf. Neumann in Montesquieu 1949: 239). Presumably jokes and the incidental were of significance even before Freud but, putting that aside, among the mythmakers of the age, racist sentiments were 'commonplace', and the racial 'other' was the invariable basis for theorizing about the nature of 'man' (Marshall and Williams 1982: 212, 246). Although Long's concern was with 'the Negro', the characteristics he discovers proved remarkably invariant in accounts of other 'races'.

As a prelude to Long, we can extract the dynamics of the formation of European identity by combining contemporary perspectives. The first step, as Ferguson recognized, is 'to imagine . . . that a mere negation of all our virtues is a sufficient description of man in his original state' (Ferguson 1966: 75). Then from this 'negative state which is styled a state of nature or a state of anarchy' is derived, in the negation of it, a 'positive' state of civilized 'subjection', including the determining order of 'positive' law (Austin 1861–3: 222 – I). The operative terms which Long accorded this replete and inviolable negation were to become

standard. (For the following see Long 1774: 353–6, 377–8 – II).
'Negroes' are conceived of in negation. They are 'void of genius
. . . either inventive or imitative'. They are 'irrational', without
'foresight', and they have 'no plan or system of morality among
them':

> They seem unable to combine ideas, or pursue a chain of
> reasoning: they have no mode of forming calculations, or of
> recording events to posterity, or of communicating thoughts
> and observations by marks, characters, or delineation.

Further, 'no rules of civil polity exist among them': they are in-
human, at one with animals or even 'below brutes'. 'Their country
in most parts is one continued wilderness, beset with briars and
thorns.' Running through all this – the lack of reason, the correspondence with the animal state, the failure to order nature – is the
inability to transcend the immediate and to act on and determine
their own being, to accept and sustain a project of self-definition.
The savage does not, in Shakespeare's astonishingly percipient
terms, 'know [its] own meaning', nor can it 'endow [its] purposes
with words that made them known' (*The Tempest* 1, ii, 356–8).
Neither action nor motivation can be constant or constructive.
'Negroes,' says Long, are 'lazy, deceitful, thievish, addicted to all
kinds of lust . . . devoted to all kinds of superstition.' Each of these
characteristics, as we shall see, become monuments to contrary
European qualities. The repertoire is extended in the fantasies of
others among the enlightened who envision savages and even
once admired civilizations as stagnant or inert, only capable of
acting out of mindless habit (custom) or caprice. The crowning
point for Long is that, despite the vastness and variety of Africa, 'a
general uniformity' of such attributes 'runs through all these
various regions of people', thereby showing them to be intrinsically different and inferior.

The beauty and necessity of this negative mode of forming
identity is that the subject is not presented in limited terms that
would contradict its equation with the universal. Even its seemingly
limiting virtues of moderation and lawfulness correspond to transcendent harmony and order. There is literally no need for Long
to account for the European in his supposed history since the
European is the active representation of the ethereal and pervasive
air within which all circumstance exists. Like glimpses of God,
Europeans are occasionally discerned in their works which Long

sees in contrast to savage incapacities as 'surely no other than the result of innate vigour and energy of the mind, inquisitive, inventive, and hurrying on with a divine enthusiasm to new attainments'. There was some small recognition of limits to European splendour in the use made of other European inventions, those of the 'noble savage' and an original state uncorrupted by such emblems of civilization as administrative efficiency and the rule of law (Ferguson 1966: 221–2). But even in these accounts, if sometimes as a matter of regret, the European remained the transcendent, ordering centre of the world. The perception of limits was to assume more challenging dimensions when, toward the end of Enlightenment, 'man' becomes a finite object of the sciences. This story is taken up in the next chapter.

The transcendent, encompassing character of European identity inhabits and secures the ways in which it is formed. The Enlightened, to borrow their motto, dared to know but to know only so much as would confirm European identity. 'It is not at all to be wonder'd', says Locke, 'that *History* gives us but a very little account of Men, *that lived together in the State of Nature*' (Locke 1965: 378 – para. 101 – his emphasis). The main problem for Locke is the absence of contemporary records. We can nonetheless be assured of the state of nature through such feats of reason – the reason Locke was so concerned to establish – as this:

> And if we may not suppose *Men* ever to have been *in the State of Nature*, because we hear not much of them in such a State, we may as well suppose the Armies of *Salmanasser*, or *Xerxes* were never Children, because we hear little of them, till they were Men and imbodied in Armies.
>
> (Locke 1965: 378 – para. 101 – his emphasis)

The massive assumption here of an intrinsic 'man' and of an ability to trace man to a single point of origin are more typically developed by Condorcet (for the following see Condorcet 1965: 195–6). 'We are obliged to guess', says Condorcet, how the 'first degrees of improvement' were attained. In this 'we can have no other guide than an investigation of the development of our faculties'. We are, however, aided by 'the history of the several societies that have been observed in almost every intermediate state,' even 'though we can follow no individual one'. Indeed, 'it is necessary to select' facts from the histories 'of different nations, and at the same time compare and combine them, to form the supposed history of a single people, and delineate its progress'. Within these epochal assumptions there was a refinement, instanced here by Goguet: 'We may judge of the state of the ancient world for some time after the deluge, by the condition of the greatest part of the new world when it was first discovered' (see Meek 1976: 21).

All this called for a large disregard of contrary evidence. The contemporary absence of knowledge cannot be an adequate excuse. Knowledge readily available was not used. The evidence relied on became increasingly threadbare and perfunctory as this body of thought 'developed'. Knowledge that would undermine it was ignored. A copious evidence showed, for example, that the savages were not savage (e.g. Axtell 1985: chapter 13). Hodgen puzzles over:

> why identifications of contemporary savagery with classical antiquity, or with old phases of other historical cultures, should ever have been made at all. So much is certain: it was not because of the validity of the correspondences cited . . . . The number of plausible likenesses elicited . . . were at best relatively few and usually trivial . . . [and] they were offset, and the conclusions derived from them were neutralized, by an overwhelming body of divergences which were seldom mentioned, much less assembled for comparison of relative proportions.
>
> (Hodgen 1964: 354–5)

This was not simply a disregard of challenging evidence. Such evidence was also re-cast. For example, the identification of 'native North American cultures' with stasis was in part 'maintained despite the discovery of powerful evidence to the contrary' but when some ability of these cultures to change was recognized, this was attributed to exterior influence (Trigger 1985: 51, 65). In short, the mythic inviolability of that 'other' against which European identity is formed was secured by elevating some kinds of knowledge and suppressing others.

In an Enlightened perspective, this line of criticism is beside the point. Since 'man's critical mind reflected the supposedly clear and rational laws of the universe' (Mosse 1978: 5), it could hardly be expected to defer to mere evidence. In its unbounded reach, it ordered and gave validity to evidence. With the ordering of things, their natures are evoked and fixed in their classification in difference (Foucault 1970: 138). Classification was, at least initially, through visual observation (Foucault 1970: 132). With the classification of races, dramatic, visible features were singled out and then massively generalized. Outward features became the signs of inner characteristics and capacities. When so equipped, the classifying gaze could produce order in hierarchical series. The medieval religious notion of the Great Chain of Being was not dissipated in a secular light but took on a fresh relevance in accounting for hierarchical racial division. Enlightened concern with the chain tended to focus on a few of the links (see Lovejoy 1966: 181). Thus, in a variant of that concern, an English adaptation of Camper's anatomy could trace the 'regular gradation from the white European down through the human species to the brute creation, from which it appears that in those particulars wherein mankind excel brutes, the European excels the African' (see Thomas 1984: 136).

As a myth of origin, this kind of story left a large hiatus. Given common origins for the savage and for the European, how were they now so radically different? For much of the eighteenth century the evidence was sought by such as Montesquieu and Bouffon in enviromental terms. A common view was that extremes – exemplified by the 'Hottentot' at one end of the known world and the 'Lapp' at the other – set racially inferior people apart from the moderate European raised in the middling, temperate zone. Strictly, the tenets of the environmentalists were contrary to racism. If racial characteristics varied with environment, climate being the most recognized influence, then a change of environment would result in a change in characteristics. These could not then be attended with that intractability which racism requires. But racism prevailed. Environmental influences served to create enduring difference or to reinforce divisions peremptorily arrived at. Simple and enormously encompassing classifications of races transcended the greatest diversity of environments experienced by people within them. In the end, environment could not provide an answer to what, despite common origins, was the difference between the savage and the European but it did provide the basis of an answer.

The grand solution settled on in the second half of the eighteenth century was the idea of progress or betterment. The notion of movement or progression in society was itself hardly a new one. In the seventeenth century, to take matters no further back, it was usual to associate the variety of people with their dispersal and progressive decline, following some original unity. This decline included the gradual loss of law and civilization. Sir Matthew Hale described such a decline, relating it to the effects of environment in *The Primitive Origination of Mankind*, a work whose continuing fame has not matched that of his contribution to law (Hale 1677: 195–7, 200–1). In the eighteenth century the hold of degeneration itself declined and the direction of movement of societies tended to be reversed with the discovery that Greeks and Romans as forebears of the European had been savages much like the Indians. So some, at least, could change and progress. 'It is in their present condition, that we are to behold, as in a mirror, the features of our progenitors' (Ferguson 1966: 80). Environment, especially as a 'mode of subsistence', now provided a basis for this change. Racial difference was linked, notably in the Scottish Enlightenment, with a vague idea of the progress of societies conceived in varying successive stages of material production – the most widely accepted becoming the hunting, the pastoral, the agricultural and the commercial. Although a matter of progression and improvement, this succession of stages was not seen as the result of some singular dynamic akin to evolution. The impetus for racially superior people to move from one stage to another was almost as varied as the diverse speculative and natural histories that accounted for it. These histories often showed as well that any such impetus could not be general for they revealed to the enlightened that there were those who did not progress and who were naturally and fixedly inferior. The mere persistence of backwardness was enough to establish its intractability. To make possible a progression beyond inferior states, each stage in the series supplanted that which went before it. Yet the civilized did harbour traces of a savage origin that had yet to be tamed: the savage passions or the dispositions of women and children, for example.

I have already indicated that the absence or contrary nature of evidence was no restraint on the imperial judgements of Enlightenment. Theorists of progress benefited greatly from that absence of restraint. It seems that the more the enlightened dared the less they needed to know. Despite their continuing hold in the West, the stories of progressive stages have never even remotely approximated to the most tolerant conditions of historical en-

THE MYTHOLOGY OF MODERN LAW

quiry, except for those recent attributions of fiction to history itself. I will now recount this tale of racism and enlightened thought in terms of the mythology of modern law.

LAW AND SAVAGERY

Despite its rejection of antiquity and its claims to total originality, the Enlightenment often re-patterned old mythic themes, making them its own. In one such theme, law is contrasted fundamentally with the savage state. For example, having left the enchantment of the Lotus-Eaters with understandably 'downcast hearts', Ulysses and his company:

> came to the land of the Cyclops race, arrogant lawless beings who leave their livelihood to the deathless gods and never use their own hands to sow or plough . . . . They have no assemblies to debate in, they have no ancestral ordinances; they live in arching caves on the tops of high hills, and the head of each family heeds no other, but makes his own ordinances for wife and children.
>
> (Shewring trans. 1980: 101 – Book IX)

As we shall see, many elements of the mythic origins of modern law are compressed into this description – the lawless nature of the savage, the emergence of law being associated with agriculture, the equation of law and sociality in contrast to the solitary state of the savage or the savage family. It was indeed common among the Greeks and Romans to identify an uncivilized or wild state with the absence of law (Kelley 1984b: 620 – chapter I; White 1978: 165). For the medieval world, exotic peoples were often monsters who did not have the capacity to follow the law because they lacked human form (see Goldberg forthcoming: chapter 1).

'In the beginning all the World was *America*' (Locke 1965: 343 – his emphasis). As a source of savage origins, the Americas remained predominant until well into the period of Enlightenment – until, that is, they were displaced as the main location of European imperial expansion. The 'discovery' of the Americas almost immediately produced a profoundly ambivalent European regard of the Indian which was to become characteristic. The Indians were wild, promiscuous, propertyless and lawless (White 1978: 186–7). Or they inhabited a 'golden worlde without toyle . . . wherein men lyved symplye and innocentlye without enforcement of lawes, without quarrelying, judges, and libelles' (see Hodgen 1964: 371). Admiration tended to decline with the intensity of aggressive European settlement. Montaigne's essay 'Of Cannibals' from the late sixteenth century was a greatly influential marker of this change (Montaigne: 1978). Although he was not without admiration for their uncorrupted state and sceptical of their disparagement by others, Montaigne's humanism ultimately accommodates the Indians in negative contrast with the civilized state. They were typified by lacks – of law, government, husbandry, and much else. Montaigne also saw the Indians as exemplars of a general state of savagery. At about the same time, this state of savagery came to be widely viewed as a general prelude to 'civil society', the main instances continuing to be the savages of the New World 'dispersed like wild beasts, lawlesse and naked' (see Hodgen 1964: 468). Comparisons were increasingly drawn between the once savage state of the Greeks and the Romans and that of the inhabitants of the Americas: 'living onely by hunting . . . without tilled landes, without cattel, without King, Law, God, or Reason' (see Meek 1976: 48–9), or 'ni foi, ni loi, ni roi' – once the virtues of a Golden Age but then a derogatory catchcry of early French explorers and settlers in North America, one to be put against the civilized condition of 'one king, one law, one faith'.

With the advent of Enlightenment these elements and more were wrought into a mythic charter by Hobbes, the 'demon-king of modernity' (cf. Tuck 1989: 102. I draw on Hobbes 1952, Introduction and chapters 13, 15, 17, 18, 26–7). Through a primal covenant between 'men':

> is created that great LEVIATHAN called a COMMON-WEALTH, or STATE (in Latin, CIVITAS), which is but an artificial man, though of greater stature and strength than the natural . . . . The pacts and covenants, by which the parts of this body politic were at first made, set together, and united, resemble that *fiat*, or the *Let us make man*, pronounced by God in the Creation.
>
> (Hobbes 1952: 47 – his emphasis)

Although this Leviathan is but a 'mortal god' (Hobbes 1952: 100), it is not restrained by mortal attributes. The binding and bonding covenant may no longer issue from the godhead but it is still attended with a mythic transcendence, inviolability and persistence. The resulting Commonwealth and its representative, the

73

sovereign, are coequally imbued with these sacred qualities. The foundational terms in which a person enters into the covenant are taken to be:

> I authorise and give up my right of governing myself to this man, or to this assembly of men, on this condition; that thou give up thy right to him, and authorise all his actions in like manner.
>
> (Hobbes 1952: 100)

Hobbes proceeds with formidable rigour to secure this pact and its creations, the Commonwealth and the sovereign, against any change or possibility of legitimate disturbance. To take just one line of argument:

> They that have already instituted a Commonwealth, being thereby bound by covenant to own the actions and judgements of one, cannot lawfully make a new covenant amongst themselves to be obedient to any other, in anything whatsoever, without his permission. And therefore, they that are subjects to a monarch cannot without his leave cast off monarchy and return to the confusion of a disunited multitude; nor transfer their person from him that beareth it to another man, or other assembly of men: for they are bound, every man to every man, to own and be reputed author of all that he that already is their sovereign shall do and judge fit to be done.
>
> (Hobbes 1952: 101)

The commitment to Leviathan is total and interminable. It is attended with the mystical union of subjects within the Commonwealth. They are taken up into the sacred realm in which they mythically participate. In being 'the author of' the Commonwealth, the subject becomes comprehensively committed to all actions of the sovereign 'as if they were his own'; subjects are thus inextricably bound: 'to him that beareth their person' – 'none of his subjects, by any pretence of forfeiture, can be freed from his subjection' (Hobbes 1952: 100–1). Ultimately, this sovereignty is the 'soul' of Leviathan: 'giving life and motion to the whole body' (1952: 47).

Hobbes proceeds to erect law in the same dimension as sovereignty. He is concerned with 'law in general', his 'design being not to show what is law here and there, but what is *law*':

'none can make laws but the Commonwealth, because our sub-jection is to the Commonwealth only', and since the sovereign is the representative of the Commonwealth 'the sovereign is the sole legislator' (1952: 130 – his emphasis). It is the 'authority of the legislator' which gives to laws a mythic persistence, which enables them to 'continue to be laws' (1952: 131). Law takes form as a 'command' of the sovereign 'addressed to one . . . obliged to obey him' (1952: 130). The moral 'laws of nature' cannot be 'properly law' until they take form as such a command (1952: 131). This command theory was to become the predominant notion in English jurisprudence but it did involve an immediate problem in that people have to know of commands in order to obey them. Hence, the command of the Commonwealth is law only to those who have means to take notice of it. 'Over natural fools, children or madman there is no law, no more than over brute beasts' (1952: 132). But if law were to be dependent on popular knowledge, this could undermine the whole edifice of authority. With unchar-acteristic equivocation, Hobbes opts largely, and understandably, for the maxim that ignorance of the law is no excuse (1952: 139). This troubling popular element of law is pursued later.

What could be the impetus or force impelling the absolute and eternal transfer of power to a mortal god? Such impetus or force comes from a negative necessity. 'Our natural passions' are in-compatible with political society: they put us in opposition to each other in 'a war as is of every man against every man' (Hobbes 1952: 85). Given this and given the rough equality of physical and mental ability among 'men', it is only through deterrence that relations between humans can emerge and they can only be crude and precarious. For anything more, a superordinate power is needed. There can be no peace 'without subjection': 'men have no pleasure (but on the contrary a great deal of grief) in keeping company where there is no power able to overawe them' (1952: 85, 99). Such a power has to be sustained – it has to make the covenant 'constant and lasting' – for without its persistence there would be a reversion to 'the condition of war', to a chaotic pre-creation, a 'return to the confusion of a disunited multitude' and 'to the sword' (1952: 100–3).

It may peradventure be thought there was never such a time nor condition of war as this; and I believe it was never generally so, over all the world: but there are many places of

America, except the government of small families, the con-
cord whereof dependeth on natural lust, have no government at all, and live at this day in that brutish manner.

(Hobbes 1952: 87–8)

The American Indian and a general invocation of savage 'places,
where men have lived by small families' provide the only
(supposedly) tangible bases of this pre-creation (Hobbes 1952:
99). Hobbes intends the American instance to be universalized,
even if 'it was never generally so', at least to the extent that 'where
there were no common power to fear' some such state would
prevail (1952: 86). He affirms the similarity of that brutish state
with the absence of a feared 'common power' when peaceful
government comes 'to degenerate into a civil war' (1952: 86). He
also invokes the antagonistic condition existing between 'kings
and persons of sovereign authority' (1952: 86). Neither of these
instances is developed, and neither would long stand comparison
with the primordial chaos provided by the simple savage, yet
Hobbes does clearly intend them to be contemporary equivalents
of the negating savagery that still lies below and that results from
an absence of overarching order. In short, 'from this very negation
is derived the positive content of the law of the land in its unconditional and unlimited validity' (Cassirer 1955: 19).

The savage state provides more than the force creating and
sustaining law and political society. It is also a specular repository
of the virtues mythically attributed to high civilizations:

Whatsoever therefore is consequent to a time of war, where
every man is enemy to every man, the same is consequent to
the time wherein men live without other security than what
their own strength and their own invention shall furnish
them withal. In such condition there is no place for industry,
because the fruit thereof is uncertain: and consequently no
culture of the earth; no navigation, nor use of the commod-
ities that may be imported by sea; no commodious building;
no instruments of moving and removing such things as
require much force; no knowledge of the face of the earth;
no account of time; no arts; no letters; no society; and which
is worst of all, continual fear, and danger of violent death;
and the life of man, solitary, poor, nasty, brutish, and short.

(Hobbes 1952: 87)

To this catalogue of negatives there are two which need to be added more specifically. These assume a close relation in a period of Enlightenment. One is the absence of property, something which Hobbes often adverts to. In the savage state there can be no security of possession and expectation: 'there be no propriety, no dominion, no *mine* and *thine* distinct; but only that to be every man's that he can get, and for so long as he can keep it' (1952: 86 – his emphasis). The other negative is the absence of law: 'where there is no common power, there is no law' and a law cannot 'be made till they have agreed upon the person that shall make it' (1952: 88).

Hobbes is the mythmaker of the tradition of overwhelming order, including its equivalent in law, legal positivism. What comes after could be seen as more or less elaborate footnotes to Hobbes's *Leviathan*. Knowledge continued to flow from the Americas of people 'without subordination, law, or form of government', joined increasingly with efforts 'to civilize this barbarism, to render it susceptible of laws' (Axtell 1985: 50). Such knowledge came to be generalized into that of an original, savage state. By the early eighteenth century, says Stein, 'the usual explanation of the origin of the state, or "civil society", as it was called, began by postulating an original state of nature, in which primitive man lived on his own. He had few social relationships with other men, and was subject to neither government nor law' (Stein 1980: 1). The 'secularized' natural law of Enlightenment was in part based on the negative reflection of this state, on what was said to be common to those nations said to be civilized (Stein 1980: 4). The monumental classifications in nature revealed by Linnaeus in 1735, after God had 'suffered him to peep into His own secret cabinet', definitively related types of *homo sapiens* to types of regulation, or lack of it: the American was regulated by custom, the European governed by laws, the Asiatic by opinion and the African by caprice (see Hodgen 1964: 425). No less influentially, Montesquieu attributed governing 'causes' to groups of people in a more sociological way, savages being dominated by nature and climate, the Japanese by laws, and so on (Montesquieu 1949: 293–4). The minority tradition of seeing the savage vices as virtues persisted. Rousseau on the whole thought it a good, if irretrievably lost, thing to have 'no society but that of the family, no laws but those of nature' (see Meek 1976: 86). With a modernist versatility worthy of the creator of Rameau's nephew, Diderot could, on site as it were, extol the

Tahitians for following their natural, especially sexual, inclinations and for not being constrained by laws; yet when closer to the Western tradition he declaims – passionately – 'the laws, the laws; there is the sole barrier that one can erect against the passions of men' (Diderot 1950; Bloch and Bloch 1980: 37; Riley 1986: 203). Even Ferguson – who censured an emerging modernity so perci- piently in his *Essay on the History of Civil Society* of 1767 and who so admired the savagery it displaced, at least in its Scottish location – saw the 'rude nations' as ultimately restrained and inferior through want of 'subordination' in a 'system of laws' and 'per- petual command' (Ferguson 1966: 121).

For the myth of law, the longest footnote to Hobbes is that provided by John Austin. It is a considerable chronological leap now to 1832 when Austin's *The Province of Jurisprudence Determined* was first published to only modest success. It is an even longer leap to the position of dominance which this work assumed and for long retained in English jurisprudence from the later nineteenth century. But Austin is very close to Hobbes and to the tradition of transcendent order. The reduced Austin lodged in English juris- prudence is well-nigh indistinguishable from Hobbes. This much is immediately evident in Austin's initial announcement that law is a command of a political superior to a political inferior (Austin 1861–3: 1, 5 – I). This 'superiority . . . is styled sovereignty', and it entails 'the relation of sovereignty and subjection': an exclusive and independent sovereignty accorded general and habitual obedience is necessary for 'political society' and law to exist (1861–3: 170–3, 179 – I). And 'in every society political and independent, the actual positive law is a creature of the actual sovereign' (1861–3: 313 – II). Although Austin does not follow Hobbes in the concentrated care devoted to foundations, the sole base evoked for his structure is savagery and it is frequently evoked. Austin draws on both a general and existent state of savagery and the 'imaginery case' of a 'solitary savage' which he takes 'the liberty of borrowing from . . . Dr. Paley' (1861–3: 82 – I. The borrowing could be Paley 1828 (1785): 4–5). This solitary savage was 'a child abandoned in the wilderness immediately after its birth, and growing to the age of manhood in estrangement from human society' (1861–3: 82 – I). As such, it could not be a 'social man', would not appreciate the necessity of property, would be in total conflict with 'his' fellows, and hence 'the ends of government and law would be defeated' (1861–3: 85 – I). The savage 'mind' is 'unfurnished' with certain notions essential for society: these 'involve the notions of political society; of supreme government; of positive law; of legal right; of legal duty; of legal injury' (1861–3: 85 – I). Austin also discovers and adverts often to a general state of savagery which he calls 'natural society' as opposed to 'political society' and which is illustrated by 'the savage . . . societies which live by hunting or fishing in the woods or on the coasts of New Holland' and by those 'which range in the forests and plains of the North American continent' (1861–3: 184 – I).

> A natural society, a society in a state of nature, or a society independent but natural, is composed of persons who are connected by mutual intercourse, but are not members, sovereign or subject, of any society political. None of the persons who compose it lives in the positive state which is styled a state of subjection: or all the persons who compose it live in the negative state which is styled a state of independence.
>
> (Austin 1861–3: 176 – I)

This negative state has none of the robust virtue of, say, Ferguson's unsubordinated Scottish Highlanders. Being a state of nature, it is completely wild and lawless (1861–3: 9 – II), and even if it were not:

> Some, moreover, of the positive laws obtaining in a political community, would probably be useless to a natural society which had not ascended from the savage state. And others which might be useful even to such a society, it probably would not observe; inasmuch as the ignorance and stupidity which had prevented its submission to political government, would probably prevent it from observing every rule of conduct that had not been forced upon it by the coarsest and most imperious necessity.
>
> (Austin 1861–3: 258 – II)

Although it is the savage which in 'negative' terms gives content to the 'political' and gives content to law, Austin does take most eloquent account of a domestic challenge to order which might seem to provide a foundation in addition to savagery, the challenge posed by 'the poor and the ignorant', especially in their misguided propensity to 'break machinery, or fire barns and corn ricks, to the end of raising wages, or the rate of parish relief' (1861–3: 62 – I). This affliction is attributed to their ignorance of the imperative good of property and capital. Its cure lies in a full appreciation of the principles of utilitarian ethics, particularly of the Malthusian variety: 'if they adjusted their numbers to the demand for their labour, they would share abundantly, with their employers, in the blessings' of property (1861–3: 62 – I). Unlike the 'stupid' savage who can only respond to the imperatives of the inexorable (Austin 1861–3: 258 – II), 'the multitude . . . can and will' come to 'understand these principles' (1861–3: 60 – I). This will be merely a boon to the law – 'an enlightened people were a better auxiliary to the judge than an army of policemen' (1861–3: 63 – I). Law is not eventually affected since such things can be resolved in terms of personal knowledge and morals. It is only the irredeemable savage which provides the ultimate limiting case against which law is constituted. One final point is needed to complete the comparison with Hobbes. As we saw, if law were a command, people needed to know of the command in order to follow it. This requirement introduced a dangerous popular element into Hobbes's scheme of things. Austin agonizes less over this and simply adopts the maxim: 'ignorance of the law is no excuse': 'if ignorance of law were admitted as a ground of exemption, the Courts would be involved in questions which it were scarcely possible to solve, and which would render the administration of justice next to impracticable' (1861–3: 171 – II). In all, the enlightening of the people can only be an aid to making existent law more effective. It cannot be intrinsic to law. Unlike the elimination of savagery, it cannot be allowed as a condition of law's existence.

Nothing could more aptly reveal the mythic nature of this commanding law than the effrontery of welding it to order in times of its infliction of massive disorder. In the increasing effort to subordinate the Indians, to 'reduce them to civility', law and order were constantly combined not just in opposition to but as a means of subduing the 'disordered and riotous' savages in their state of lawless 'anarchy', but often with the realization that they may, after all, remain uncontrollable and unpredictable (Axtell 1985: 136–8). This scenario precisely reverses what was the case.

European intervention was freighted with the deathly disordering of an already and subtly ordered situation – a situation which, for the European, 'was literally unthinkable' (Axtell 1985: 137). Nonetheless, this association of law with order, security and regularity rapidly became general and obvious, the violence associated with the establishment of law and order assuming insignificance in the immeasurability of the violence and disorder of savagery (see e.g. Ferguson 1966: 221–2; Meek 1976: 204). For Austin, 'general security' and a 'general feeling of security' are 'the principal ends of political society and law' and these are the antithesis of that 'negative state which is styled a state of nature or a state of anarchy' (1861–3: 84, 122 – I). The very mind of the savage, as we saw, is 'unfurnished' with the notions of political society and law (Austin 1861–3: 85 – I). Like the Cyclops, 'his thinking is lawless, unsystematic and rhapsodical' (Adorno and Horkheimer 1979: 65). This contrasts essentially with 'the uniformity of conduct produced by an imperative law' (Austin 1861–3: 159 – I). The colonial situation provides another monumental instance of law initiating and sustaining pervasive disorder even in the pursuit of its pretence to secure order. An abundance of instances can also be found in the more domestic European settings where modern law explicitly confronted and sought to undermine an existing order which was often, in the process, rendered in the terms created for savagery and barbarian despotisms. As a mode of modernity, law was an instrument of far-reaching change integral to the 'tearing down and building up' (Cassirer 1955: ix). But no matter what its visitations of disorder and no matter what the distance between its practice and the perfection of its order, law remains mythically inviolable in its intrinsic equation with order.

Disorder on law's part cannot, then, be located in law itself. The sources of disorder must exist outside of law – in the eruptions and disruptions of untamed nature or barely contained human passion against which an ordering law is intrinsically set. The savage was the concentration of these dangers and the constant and predominant want of the savage was order. Savages had 'no skill of submission' (see Axtell 1985: 271). Ferguson admired them for their lawless minds, for being unable to 'accept commands' and for being opposed to 'subordination', something which could be taken as an exact counterpoint to Austin's idea of law (Ferguson 1966: 84).

I will now explore this state of savagery in its opposition to the order of law. A particular and indicative obsession of colonist and *philosophe* alike was the lack of fixity in savage life. Indians could not begin to be civilized until they were in a 'fixed condition of life': 'Their Nature is so volatile, they can few or none of them be brought to fix to a trade' (see Axtell 1985: 141, 160). Lacking resolution themselves, they could not project it onto a world: they 'have none of the spirit, industry, and perseverance necessary in those who *subdue* a wilderness' (see Axtell 1985: 149 – emphasis in the original). With 'primitive common ownership', declared Grotius, men were content 'to feed on the spontaneous products of the earth, to dwell in caves' (see Meek 1976: 15). They did not constructively tame nature. What Grotius was thus content to learn from 'sacred history', Locke arrived at with no history at all. The savage was a wanderer or related to land in an indefinite communal way, not sufficiently 'removed from the common state Nature placed it in' (Locke 1965: 329 – para. 27). In either capacity, the savage had no sufficiently fixed relation to things to support a legal right to them. Property was the basis of law. In the state of nature, Austin confirmed: 'men . . . have no legal rights' (1861–3: 9 – II). The convenient ignorance of the European thence found a 'void' and 'wilderness' in savage climes, a lack of fixed position and tenure, such as to justify and even require the assertion of an 'exclusive right' and the acquiring of 'sovereignty' over them – borrowing here the sentiments of de Vattel, 'perhaps the most widely read of all eighteenth-century authorities on international law' (Curtin 1971: 42–3). For Vattel and for this so-called international law, it is not simply a matter of when 'a Nation finds a country inhabited and without an owner, it may lawfully take possession of it' but also a Nation may likewise occupy a territory 'in which are to be found only wandering tribes whose small numbers can not populate the whole country', since 'their uncertain occupancy of these vast regions can not be held as a real and lawful taking of possession' (Vattel 1971: 44–5). Inadequate production as well as inadequate peopling justified European appropriation:

> For I aske whether in the wild woods and uncultivated waste of America left to Nature, without any improvement, tillage or husbandry, a thousand acres will yield the needy and wretched inhabitants as many conveniencies of life as ten acres of equally fertile land doe in Devonshire where they are well cultivated?
> (Locke 1965: 336 – para. 37)

(Indeed, for Locke, the absence of a fixed, cultivating relation to land accounted for the lack of reason itself (see Hulme 1990: 30).) In short, and in mythic terms, settlement 'is equivalent to an act of Creation' (Eliade 1965: 10).

Law becomes generally and integrally associated with the mythic settling of the world – with its adequate occupation and its bestowal on rightful holders, the Occidental 'possessors and builders of the earth' (Levinas 1979: 46). Blackstone provides a most significant account in his *Commentaries on the Laws of England*, first published between 1765 and 1769 (and amended by Blackstone up to the sixteenth edition of 1825 which I use here). Although it is customary to portray Blackstone as the supreme systematizer and popularizer of English law, his originality has been denied more than extolled (cf. Lieberman 1989: 31–3; Milsom 1981). Unfair as this assessment may be for his work in general, what is important about his account of law and the settlement of the world is that it is, style apart, so unremarkable. It reflects and encapsulates the thought of the age and brings it to bear on the creation of law. It is to be found at the outset of the second volume of the *Commentaries* dealing with property. 'There is', he begins, 'nothing which so generally strikes the imagination, and engages the affections of mankind, as the right of property' (Blackstone 1825: 1 – II). He then sets out 'the original and foundation' of the right of property, proceeding by way of *Genesis* and the pervasive dominion 'the all-bountiful Creator gave to man' to the 'state of primeval simplicity: as may be collected from the manners of many American nations when first discovered by the Europeans; and from the antient method of living among the first Europeans themselves' (1825: 2–3 – II). Property was then held in common and the only personal element in property was the holding of things for immediate use. 'But when mankind increased in number, craft, and ambition, it became necessary to entertain conceptions of more permanent dominion' (1825: 4 – II). The result was first a transition from 'the wild and uncultivated' nations to a pastoral existence when the 'world by degrees grew more populous'; then it 'became necessary' to resort to 'the art of agriculture' and for this private property was found to be essential:

> Had not therefore a separate property in lands, as well as moveables, been vested in some individuals, the world must have continued a forest, and men have been mere animals of prey; which, according to some philosophers, is the genuine state of nature . . . . Necessity begat property: and in order to insure that property, recourse was had to civil society, which

brought along with it a long train of inseparable concomit-
ants; states, government, laws.

(Blackstone 1825: 5, 7 – II)

This was and remains a common story. Whether or not impelled
by an increasing population, the joint arrival of agriculture and
property – property not just as things but as the great figure of
settlement and order – requires a complex and more intense regulation than the episodic assertions called for in the nomadic or
even in the pastoral state; what is required is an explicit, per-
manently sustained ordering that is law (see Meek 1976: 93, 102–4;
Stein 1980: 28, 33–6). In the result, the paradigm of law corresponds to the property relation. Blackstone secured in English law
a structure in which the person engages in formal action which
affects things or 'the field of acquisition' (Kelley 1984b: 624 –
chapter I). This is but a ritualized form of how Occidental social
and imperial action relates to the world. Sir Matthew Hale, evoked
by Blackstone as an ancestor, had already rendered 'man's'
general relation to nature in quasi-legal terms whereby 'Man was
invested with power, authority, right, dominion, trust and care'
(Hale 1677: 370).

The relation of law to property and sustained order had been
refined in advance of Blackstone by Locke. Even if less dire than it
was for Hobbes, the state of nature in Locke's view was still dangerous and uncertain. These defects were cured only by entering
into a political or civil society marked by law:

> Those who are united into one Body, and have a common
> establish'd Law and Judicature to appeal to, with Authority to
> decide controversies between them, and punish Offenders,
> *are in Civil Society* one with another; but those who have no
> such common Appeal, I mean on Earth, are still in the state
> of Nature, each being, where there is no other, Judge for
> himself, and Executioner; which is, as I have before shew'd it,
> the perfect *state of Nature.*
>
> (Locke 1965: 367 – para. 87 – his emphasis)

The 'Civiliz'd part of Mankind', in contrast, is characterized by
'positive laws' (1965: 331 – para. 30). Then, most famously, Locke
ties that entry into political society with the securing of property,
fusing central, sovereign command with the order of settlement.
'The great and *chief end* therefore, of Mens uniting into Common-

wealths, and putting themselves under Government, *is the Preserva-tion of their Property*' (1965: 395 – para. 124 – his emphasis). He immediately proceeds to delineate the rule of law as a response to 'many things wanting . . . in the state of Nature', as a response, at its most general, to the chaos of merely individual assertions of passion and self-interest:

> *First,* There wants an *establish'd,* settled, known *Law,* received and allowed by common consent to be the Standard of Right and Wrong, and the common measure to decide all Con-troversies between them . . . . *Secondly,* In the State of Nature there wants a *known and indifferent Judge,* with Authority to determine all differences according to the established Law . . . *Thirdly,* In the state of Nature there often wants *Power* to back and support the Sentence when right, and to *give* it due *Execution.*
>
> (Locke 1965: 396 – paras. 124–6 – his emphasis)

This new law is characterized by a unifying strength. Adam Smith, in his *Lectures on Jurisprudence,* finds that with the society of hunters for disputes outside the family 'the whole community . . . interferes to make up the difference: which is ordinarily all the length they go, never daring to inflict what is properly called punishment' (1978: 201). 'Barbarous nations' had weak governments unable, for example, to enforce the death penalty for murder, 'the only proper punishment' and the one inflicted in 'strong', 'civilized nations' (1978: 106, 476). This capacity is elevated in those terms of sovereignty which were earlier traced to Hobbes. To take a famed definition from Austinian jurisprudence:

> If a *determinate* human superior, *not* in a habit of obedience to a like superior, receive *habitual* obedience from the *bulk* of a given society, that determinate superior is sovereign in that society, and the society (including the superior) is a society political and independent.
>
> (Austin 1861–3: 170 – I – his emphasis)

Although this position is ultimately sustained in terms of strength, the stronger state does not incorporate the feeble since 'there is neither a *habit* of command on the part of the former, nor a *habit* of obedience on the part of the latter' (Austin 1861–3: 173 – I – his emphasis). Each retains its distinct force, its distinct centre of power and, hence, its own determinacy: 'no indeterminate party

can command expressly or tacitly, or can receive obedience or
submission: . . . no indeterminate body is capable of corporate
conduct, or is capable, as a body, of positive or negative de-
portment' (1861–3: 175 – I). 'Every law properly so called flows
from a *determinate* source, or emanates from a *determinate* author'
(1861–3: 120 – I – his emphasis). Austin's consolidation of the idea
of sovereignty replicates within modernity the mythic symbolism of
the ordering centre of creation. Only that which comes from the
centre has validity (Eliade 1965: 18). Law exists by virtue of its
'position' in identification with the sovereign and centre (Austin
1861–3: 2 – I). It takes on the impression of the *imago mundi*,
affirming the ordered, normal course, often by correcting deviations from that course. The creation and enforcement of any law
is a ritual reassertion of the foundational strength and ordering of
the centre (cf. Eliade 1965: 20). What is being affirmed is not just
a particular order in opposition to disorder but the very being and
force of order itself.

This order, in its originating opposition to savage chaos,
accords a unity to law transcending its diverse and contradictory
elements, thus making coherent legal order possible. Locke, as we
saw, exemplified the fusing of command with settled order – the
sovereign god with the god captured by a fixed creation – through
their common negation in the savage state. Law is further captured
in order by its own subjects. Even Hobbes, who would recognize
popular participation in law only in a mythical act of self-
alienation, was discomfited by the necessity of the subject's having
to recognize the sovereign's command (1952: 39). We can approach this dimension of order by refining the disorder of simple
savagery as the foil of law. Even in 'a territory of considerable
extent', wrote Ferguson, where the inhabitants retain their
'warlike and turbulent spirit', they can be ordered by the 'bridle of
. . . barbarian despotism': and in the later eighteenth century it
became a fashion to contrast law with fickle despotisms, particularly of the oriental variety (Ferguson 1966: 103–4; and see
Marshall and Williams 1982: 140). Law was integrally part of and
endured as the civilized European order. Outside this order, there
was either the unpredictable arbitrariness of despotism or the
inconstancy and mindless hedonism of the simple savage (Ferguson 1966: 93, 95). In law, human projects could be initiated by
members of political or civil society and secured in time (see e.g.
Locke 1965: 344 – para. 50). Rousseau combined all elements of

the mix: law was needed because 'society must have activities and ends'; law also embodied and sustained what civilization had managed to inculcate so far and it dealt with those continuing assertions of nature inimical to order(Strauss and Cropsey 1972: 542–4). So, returning to Austin, law is not just a peremptory command: it is also 'a command which obliges a person or persons to a *course* of conduct' (1861–3: 15 – I). 'An imperative law or rule guides the conduct of the obliged, or is a *norma*, model, or pattern, to which their conduct conforms' (1861–3: 159 – I). Law creates enduring rights and obligations of which the pre-social savage can know nothing (1861–3: 85 – I). There is a contradiction between law as a simple command of a sovereign and law as project, model and obligation, dependent on popular support and adherence. This contradiction is also mediated through law's relation to savagery. Since in both these situations law is created as a negation of the savage state, it is created the same and unified in that essence which Enlightenment derives from origins.

LAW AND PROGRESS

Seemingly in opposition to an ordered legality, modern law also comes into being in a process of change and progression. It is not (just) a command coming from above nor is it tied fixedly to any order; rather, it responds in its constitution to change in 'society'. This part of the myth, which I now explore, is worked out in the narratives of law and progress; and the story, as we shall see, is told in such a way as to enable it to be reconciled with the imperative of order.

There are certain precursors of progress to be sketched in first. Law has to be linked to society, or distinct types of law linked to distinct 'nations', as they were called. The significant ancestor figure here seems to be Montesquieu. The 'laws' whose 'spirit' he sought cannot readily be equated with modern ideas of law but that difficulty has not obstructed his received reputation as the progenitor of the connection between law and society. Montesquieu thought that laws have or ought to have a relation to several shaping factors and 'that it should be a great chance if those of one nation suit another' (1949: 6). He enumerated a considerable number of shaping factors – climate, geography, 'principal occupation of the natives', 'the degree of liberty which the constitution will bear', religion, and so, considerably, on: 'all these together constitute what I call the Spirit of the Laws' (1949: 6–7). There were contemporaries and predecessors who made connections between law and society if of a different kind. Hobbes and Hume, among others, equated sociality with a necessary minimum legality (Hobbes 1952: chapters 14 and 15; Hume 1888: Book III parts 1–2). Given supposedly obvious circumstances of the human condition – circumstances of moderate equality of powers, moderate selfishness and moderate scarcity – the existence and civility of human society must depend 'on the strict observance' of laws securing 'the stability of possession, its transference, and the performance of promises' (Hume 1888: Book III part I – para. 6). This equation of a distinct configuration of bourgeois law with universal necessity had no more existent foundation than the assertion that everyone slept between clean sheets but it has nonetheless endured in the mythology of modern law. Neither these contributions nor that of Montesquieu sought to relate different laws to different societies in a scheme or sequence of progression. Montesquieu, however, did outline one influence on law which was to prove momentous in its development by the chroniclers of progression: that is the

> very great relation to the manner in which the several nations procure their subsistence. There should be a code of laws of a much larger extent for a nation attached to trade and navigation than for people who are content with cultivating the earth. There should be a much greater for the latter than for those who subsist by their flocks and herds. There must be a still greater for these than for such as live by hunting.
>
> (Montesquieu 1949: 275)

What is more, Montesquieu provided a way of recognizing a diversity of types of law in different settings. Law did not, in this view, simply emerge at some stage and prior to that there was non-law. Even those with the most adverse assessment of savages could, in this temper, attribute some law to them even if it be 'irrational and ridiculous': although 'laws have been justly regarded as the master-piece of human genius . . . the jurisprudence, the customs and manners of the Negroes, seem perfectly suited to the measure of their narrow intellect', including their inability to create 'regulations dictated by forsight' (Long 1774: 378 – Book III). As Long's 'scientific' assessment indicates, the linking of law and society was accompanied by an expansion of the peoples brought into contention, an expansion beyond the previously predominant concern with the American Indian. Indeed, the historical and geographic range of peoples considered by Montesquieu could be seen as a large contribution to the universal sweep which the doctrine of progress inexorably imports.

These various relations of law to societies coalesce with the invention of progress and connect law to sequential stages of progress usually conceived in terms of four modes of 'subsistence' – the hunting, the pastoral, the agricultural and the commercial (see Meek 1976). The overall trajectory of these stories remained the same as those idylls of order in which the primordial and savage gives way to the civilized life. There was a rough similarity in the numerous tales of progression but probably one of the most enduring influences was provided by Adam Smith in his *Lectures on Jurisprudence*, a work which even now silently sets the broad terms of the comparative sociology of law (Smith 1978). With the progression of societies, law for Smith increased in quantity and complexity and in its distinctness as a social form. As with many of these accounts, the advance of law was tied integrally to the progressive consolidation of property: the 'early age of hunters', as typified by the American Indians, had no property and hence few laws and an uncivilized legal system (1978: 16, 201). With the pastoral stage, people are more numerous, there is a greater division of labour, property is more extensive, and 'distinctions of rich and poor' emerge: 'permanent laws' and the expansion of authority are now needed to secure property and the rich (1978: 202, 208–9). With such 'useful inequality in the fortunes of mankind', the poor could yet be consoled because they lived in a far greater opulence than any savage prince (1978: 338, 562; see also Locke 1965: 339 – para. 41). No new foundational impetus is adduced for law's progression into the ages of agriculture and commerce but there are further changes in law. Quantitatively, there is more law and an increasingly stronger central authority. Qualitatively, the simple legal regime of the whole community which characterizes pastoralists gives way to more complex and institutionally separate forms of authority, to legislatures and regular courts (1978: 204–5). Although the procession of stages, for Smith and its other chroniclers, was serially supplanting, progression was a continuing creation, still traced back continuously to the state of savagery which remained a constant contrast and point of reference, no matter for what stage. I will now look a little more closely at the nature of this progression before bringing matters to a conclusion.

It may seem rash to depart from the admirable work of Stein (1980) and Meek (1976) showing that, for law and for the social sciences, this progression is a type of evolution. Matters seem to be more mixed and, for my purposes, more revealing. For a start, there was hardly that underlying, unitary and unifying dynamic inhabiting the progression which is usually associated with evolution. The impetus for the progression varied greatly with the different accounts of it. In some tales, progress depends on the characteristics of those who progress – 'the more industrious and discerning part of mankind', the more highly educated, or those who increase in 'craft, and ambition' (Blackstone 1825: 4; Riley 1986: 248; Stein 1980: 22). In other versions, or sometimes in the very same version, there was great emphasis on more external factors, such as the increase in population: an increase in population requires an increase in resources or an increase in resources enabled population to increase. What in one moment were consequences of progress became in another its cause, and vice versa. Thus, an increasing sociality results from an increasing population or an increasing population results from increasing sociality (see Meek 1976: 163). All of which is mixed with inspiring metaphors of the 'rise' and 'spirit' of society (Meek 1976: 5; Stein 1980: 28).

To labour such incoherence would be little better than facile because there was no coherent evolutionary dynamic involved in the progression. The contrary assertion, to borrow it from Stein, is that the thinkers in France and Scotland who developed the idea of progression 'treated the mode of subsistence as not merely one of several factors affecting the character of a society's laws but as the crucial circumstance which dictated their nature and scope', and on that basis they erected 'a scheme of development' (Stein 1980: 19). Such a notion of 'legal evolution' is presented by Stein in a careful and abundant illustration. There certainly is progression but, as we have just seen, there is no general dynamic giving it identity and effect. Something else is at work. Law is being typologically related to diverse and distinct modes of subsistence. In the 'spirit' of the times, law is identified in simplifying and classifying relation to other things, in 'a coherent pattern', as Stein describes the object of the quest (Stein, 1980: 27). Law is thus located and identified in 'the order of things', in an order that springs from within the things ordered (Foucault 1970: 209). Progression becomes a mode of tracing that identity. This can be exemplified in a quotation which Stein provides from Kames's metaphorical journey on the Nile – a Nile whose enormous and inextricable complexities are indicatively reduced to the simple progress of more straightforward domestic streams:

> When we enter upon the municipal law of any country in its present state we resemble a traveller, who crossing the Delta, loses his way among the numberless branches of the Egyptian river. But when we begin at the source and follow the current of law . . . all its relations and dependencies are traced with no greater difficulty, than are the many streams into which that magnificent river is divided before it is lost in the sea.
>
> (see Stein 1980: 26)

This sustained progression emanating from a source in savagery exists within a still foundational order. It is the story of something achieved, not of something still being achieved. What is talked of here is the perfection and completeness of law and what comes before are simply its pale precursors. The chroniclers of law and progression did not see themselves as departing from a foundational equation of law with order. The progression does not supplant the order of things and proceed to identify law as part of a pervasive and encompassing dynamic. The thought was not there to elevate a dynamic of progression into an impelling and cohering evolution. Any concern with an actual dynamic of progression was, rather, diverse, inconsistent and almost incidental.

Progression can be an elaboration of order because both are traced to the same constituting source. In 'the order of things', to find the origin of a thing is to locate its being. The opposition between the progression of law and law's order is mediated and the two are united in the origin of a primal and chaotic savagery. Both the progression and the order of law take their being in the negation or denial of this 'state of nature'. Positive law, being constituted simply in terms of what it is not, can be self-contained and self-presenced. Change becomes a refinement of legal order and contributes towards its perfection. In its being without restriction, law can now do anything. An infinite capacity for change – for law itself changing and for effecting change – is associated with order. This enviable instrument of rule is presented in more spectacularly virtuous ways as the rule of law – for law to rule, it must be able to do anything. The incredulous cannot definitively attribute limits to a law constituted in negation.

4

THE MYTHIC CONSOLIDATION OF MODERN LAW

Our civilization is characterized by the word 'progress'. Progress is its form rather than making progress being one of its features.

(Wittgenstein 1980: 7e)

THE REIGN OF FINITUDE

Towards the end of the period of Enlightenment, the sovereign subject is dethroned and there remains no one to do the work of the gods. The all-seeing, surrogate deity is subordinated in 'the sciences of man and society' to a reign of finitude. However, as we saw in chapter 2, the 'man' that emerges from this change is not just an object of knowledge, 'a creature of finitude and limits', but also a transcendent 'source of order for the totality' (Foucault 1970: 313–14). The contradiction between these two states is mythically resolved in the perfection of progression. Progression no longer simply inhabits and confirms the object as an element in its achieved state: rather, the object enters into an encompassing progression. But progression, in all its promise, also remains in the object, even if no longer bound by its achieved state. The present condition of man as an object is a harbinger of boundless being yet to be fully discovered or constructed. However, for man as a 'source of order for the totality' there can be no deferral of the demand for pure transcendence. There are no fixed points on the path of future progress at which fateful shortcomings can be marked and allowed for. The transcendence of man operates immediately and completely, creating a modern subjectivity that is all-embracing and infinitely responsive.

Progression itself and the identity of man which it informs are not teleologically specific. Progression is a transcendent, limitless realm of possibility. No matter how inspirational the process – man's heroic advance against nature, the unfolding of universal spirit – the outcome of progression is vague, potential and even uncertain. It acquires operative specificity and lends a tangible identity to man not by being a progression to but a progression from some state. What is involved here, I will argue, is a dynamic of identity in negation similar in basic ways to that presented in the last chapter. This similarity produces a continuity in myth despite the cogent perception of an epistemic break late in the period of Enlightenment (Foucault 1970). A classifying, spatial ordering of the world seems to recede and an evolutionary, temporal force seems to emerge. But there is a linking homology in the racially hierarchic succession within each system which enables a continuity in myth to be erected. This is part of the very continuity which the perception of an epistemic break confirms by being set against it. So, a myth of modernity would retrospectively see the progress invented in Enlightenment as incipient evolution although the two are radically different in their epistemic depths (Foucault 1970: 150–4).

This new epistemic scheme ushers in pervasive and inexorable change. The new sciences of life are coterminous with reality and being. They are intrinsically responsive to change and are themselves constantly changing and developing. There is no longer an order of things, a set natural law or any other enduring substrate. Yet science does not simply encounter and confirm a promiscuous or chaotic change. Science creates or 'discovers' order, even if that order is always held provisional, and it extends a unifying order presumptively to all that is yet to be discovered. (Chaos theory is somewhat of an exception to this.) The mythic resolution of the contradiction between order and change is provided in a progression which matches change, incorporating or at least orienting it in a unitary, linear and serial ordering. For social thought, the most influential form of that progression has been evolution. This influence is not confined to the application of evolutionary doctrine to society but extends to the enduring terms that evolution has bequeathed to modern social thought.

THE PERFECTION OF PROGRESS

The predominant mythmaker of evolution has of course been Darwin. It is usual to soften accounts of his work by extricating him from the misuse of his ideas by a cousin and other contemporaries. I am not immediately concerned with the extent to which Darwin's scientific work was sullied by racists and social evolutionists. Nor am I concerned with the extent to which the always uncertain idea of evolution has, in scientific terms, been qualified or undermined by later work in palaeontology and palaeoanthropology. This later work does have an oblique significance for my concerns in that the devastating specialist opposition to the idea of evolution is a testament to its persistence as myth. The denial of Darwin's culpability for the abuse of evolutionary ideas holds those ideas and Darwin as their originator (a not entirely accurate attribution) in a realm of mythic purity. The pathologies visited on evolution are thus rendered exceptional and evanescent. My argument, on the contrary, is that these supposed pathologies are intrinsic to evolution as myth and that Darwin is a sufficiently generous figure to accommodate them.

Misia Landau tells us that 'of all the stories paleo-anthropologists have told', and there are a great diversity of them, 'only Darwin's *The Descent of Man* . . . approaches the status of an authorized version' (Landau 1991: 19). Darwin had already anticipated that his account of 'the origin of species' would throw light on 'the origin of man and his history' (Darwin 1970: 458). Here now was a new genesis for man, if not at first sight a propitious one – a natural development from animal ancestry. Man was subsumed in life and subject to the same forces that created all its forms. Nonetheless a distinct humanity was extracted from the process. This involved a history hardly less speculative than the most imaginative eighteenth-century variety in which the 'descent' of man from a 'lower' form is initiated in a descent from the trees because of a supposed 'change in its manner of procuring subsistence, or some change in the surrounding conditions' (Darwin 1948: 433). The terrestrial existence proves decidedly more Hobbesian than a balmy arboreality. The challenge of this new state produces behaviour that is omnivorous, aggressive and progressive – an intriguing combination. Somewhat paradoxically, this behaviour enhances a superior propensity for social existence that resides within man or within incipient man (Darwin 1948: 478). Thence, through various psychological and mental developments, there is a transition from the animal to the human. Then there is a culminating further shift, this time from savagery to civilization.

Despite an ensuing broad consensus around this type of story, there was and remains little agreement or clarity about its effective dynamic. The diversity and even the content of propelling causes not only match those offered in eighteenth-century stories of progress but add to them with a penchant for anatomical factors. There remained nonetheless an adherence to an elevated, subsuming development. In some versions, usually considered the more scientific, this was a progression without teleology. It simply was. The effects, for example, of random mutation in a process of natural selection could, obviously, not be subordinated to a purpose or end. But the opposite view could just as readily be found: 'as natural selection works solely by and for the good of each being, all corporeal and mental endowments will tend to progress towards perfection' (Darwin 1970: 459).

We can begin with Jones's help to develop the mythic link between evolutionary progression and the individual:

> In 1866 Wallace had warned Darwin about the phrase 'Natural Selection'. He believed it would be misunderstood and that the terms 'Nature' and 'Selection' would tend to imply a directing intelligence in evolution. But to warn against a form of words is to misunderstand a fundamental intellectual and social process. The belief in Direction and Intelligence generating history would have been introduced regardless. Behind this were social pressures which required that the social order be pictured as a pattern of rational categories – in other words that society was as it was because this was the best or most reasonable way it could be. A second major characteristic was to describe society and social and racial places in it in terms of individual attributes. What social Darwinists saw in natural selection was not dispelled by Wallace's alternative title 'survival of the fittest'. The latter term neatly coincided with another of their basic premises – that social position and social action is a function of individual faculty.
>
> (Jones 1980: 143)

Darwin placed particular emphasis on the growth of 'intellectual faculties' (Darwin 1948: chapters 3 and 4). With 'natural selection', for example, we find that 'the real struggle in *The Descent of Man* occurs not between animals and men but between humans of varying intellects' (Landau 1991: 50). Darwin had already

THE MYTHOLOGY OF MODERN LAW

intimated in *The Origin of Species* that 'as the individuals of the same species come into the closest competition with each other, the struggle will be most severe between them' (Darwin 1970: 442).

The link between progression and the individual is mediated in terms of race. When addressing the advance of man from a savage to a civilized state:

> Darwin passed almost unconsciously from individual struggle and selection, to group or racial struggle and selection. . . . Human races, to Darwin, formed discrete mental and moral units based on biological difference . . . . Darwin also accepted that the races formed a mental and moral hierarchy, from the least to the most moral and intelligent.
>
> (Stepan 1982: 57)

That hierarchy, the domination of one race over another, was the outcome of evolutionary struggle between them. The result, Darwin said, depended on 'which have the best fitted organization, or instinct (i.e., intellect in man) to gain the day' (see Stepan 1982: 57). And it was the European race that had gained the day. Evolution could accommodate the competing variety within a species and provide a basis for evaluating different 'forms' within the species, 'favouring the good and rejecting the bad' (Darwin 1970: 108, 443). In *The Descent of Man*, the savage was judged frequently and severely, extending even to a preference for certain heroic simians over the 'savage who delights to torture his enemies, offers up bloody sacrifices, practises infanticide without remorse, treats his wives like slaves, knows no decency, and is haunted by the grossest superstitions' (Darwin 1948: 919–20). The terms of this superiority were similar to those in eighteenth-century myths of origin. They included the progressive domination of reason or, now, intelligence over nature and the development of social organization, and all this at the expense of inferior others who can be subordinated or displaced (e.g. Darwin 1948: 478, 1970: 445).

It may at first sight seem contradictory to talk about an evolutionary foundation for racist thought. After all, no matter how inferior, inferior races could presumably still evolve into higher positions. They could even be assisted in this by a superior race, an argument whose frequency matched the spread of formal colonization. But race finally obstructed the prospect of improvement in two ways. With one, a racism for all practical purposes admitted the prospect of improvement but deferred its achievement: to change 'ignorant and savage races', said Dickens, 'is a work which, like the progressive changes of the globe itself, requires a stretch of years that dazzles in the looking at' (see Brantlinger 1985: 174). With the other obstruction to improvement, intractable racial inferiority was seen as an outcome of evolution, not as something to be overcome by it. The two obstructions were combined in a view common in colonial situations that the 'native' could improve but only 'thus far and no further'.

These barriers to the progress of inferior races were confirmed in a race science which can only be separated in retrospect from evolutionary thought. The numberless measurements of cranial capacities and facial profiles, and the attribution of varied mental and moral characters to the supposed outcomes of these measurements, were not cranky and aberrant activities. Such things were within the mainstream of the new sciences of man and society. Robert Knox, to take an example, is usually seen as a foundational figure in race science. Accounts now of *The Races of Man*, first published in 1850, tend to mockery of its virulent racism and rampant imperialism. Fryer's admirable work does this to Knox but Darwin escapes – his theories were 'distorted' (Fryer 1988: 174–5, 181). Yet Knox, in terms that were then at the scientific forefront, connects man with 'all life' and finds him inseparable 'from the organic world'; he also anticipates key Darwinian doctrines (Knox 1862: 11, 33, 42–3). Knox did at least have the virtue of recognizing that the 'Saxon race', whilst strong and inexorable in its imperial advance, was duplicitous in its claim that such an advance was in the cause of humanity and civilization.

Even more significant is the inverse influence where race science inhabits what is taken to be mainstream science. This is not simply a matter of 'the history of racial science [being] a history of a series of accommodations of the sciences to the demands of deeply held convictions about the "naturalness" of the inequalities between human races' (Stepan 1982: xx-i). The sciences of man and society do not exist apart from these accommodations. Darwin, for one, did not see the racial theories of Spencer or even of Knox as something different to his work (see e.g. Darwin 1888: 428). Nor can the continuing influence of race and evolution in social thought be adequately contained in small but surviving intellectual fields, such as evolutionary sociology. That influence, I now argue, remains pervasive.

We could start with the paradox of Spencer. From an un-
paralleled elevation in his time, he has been relegated to a place of
transience in the history of social thought. The reasons are not
difficult to discern. His invention of social evolution and his
general transfer of biological forces to social settings were effected
in racial and, to an extent, racist terms. Groups of people and their
social institutions were placed on 'the ladder of evolution' in
accord with their race. This was the outcome of 'the struggle for
existence' in which 'lower' and 'inferior' races lost out or were
slower to advance. Inferior races were identified, in terms of the
day, as having less weight and activity in the brain or having a
sharper angle to their facial profile, and so on. They were also
identified, in terms shared with an older Occidental tradition, by
their mode of subsistence and their 'rigidity of custom' (see Haller
1975: 123–9). But Spencer was creating a new tradition, one
located in the sciences of life and one in which all was impelled or
held together by 'the general law of evolution'.

Thus, Spencer, in furthering a 'survey of the facts' which justify
the comparison of a society to a living body, finds 'that the paral-
lelism becomes the more marked the more closely it is traced'
(Spencer 1972: 61). Having described the structure of various
protozoa, he says:

> these little societies of monads, or cells, or whatever else we
> may call them, are societies only in the lowest sense: there is
> no subordination of parts among them – no organization.
> Each of the component units lives by and for itself: neither
> giving nor receiving aid. There is no mutual dependence,
> save that consequent on mere mechanical union.
>
> (Spencer 1972: 61)

He then foists these attributes onto the 'lowest' races instancing a
common choice among evolutionists for low racial status, the
so-called Bushmen (whose social organization was the antithesis of
these attributes):

> Now do we not here discern 'analogies' to the first stages of
> human societies? Among the lowest races, as the Bushmen,
> we find but incipient aggregation: sometimes single families:
> sometimes two or three families wandering about together.
> The number of associated units is small and variable; and
> their union instant. No division of labour except between the

sexes; and the only kind of mutual aid is that of joint attack or defence. We see nothing beyond an undifferentiated group of individuals, forming the germ of a society; just as in the homogenous groups of cells above described we see only the initial stage of animal and vegetable organization.

(Spencer 1972: 61)

Spencer continues in this vein, which is typically mythic in its extracting origins of society from the processes of nature, moving now beyond the relative chaos of pre-creation to more complex polyps: 'instead of such small variable groups as are formed by Bushmen, we come to the larger and more permanent groups formed by savages not quite so low, and we begin to find traces of social structure' (Spencer 1972: 61). The progression proceeds in tandem with growing sociality in a movement from nomadic to 'semi-settled' to settled societies, thence to civilization (Spencer 1972: 144–5). The general advance is mapped in terms of the increase in several dynamic factors – the scale of societies, the differentiation of social functions, cooperation and the complexity of organization and structure of social life (Spencer 1972: 62).

Is the purifying expulsion of Spencer from social thought accompanied by the expulsion of the mythology? As the terms of advance in the story he tells indicate, not at all. The mythology may have become 'whitened' but it manifestly survives, and it survives not just in particular traits such as the increasing complexity of societies but also in the operation of encompassing mythic forces that provide the origins, persistent core and impelling dynamic of society and its development. The forces are presented in vitalist narratives which tell of man's progressive domination of nature, and such. These mythic powers also imbue the constituent parts of society, providing origins and a sequenced development for such entities as the family, law and property.

In its most general effect, the modern demiurge takes a variety of forms. I will instance, doubtless with unforgivable brevity, the ancestor figures of modern social thought, Marx, Durkheim and Weber. Despite rejecting aspects of Spencer, it is Durkheim who stands closest to him. With Durkheim's famed distinction, 'mechanical solidarity' was found predominantly in primitive societies which were amorphous, communal and kin-based; whereas 'organic solidarity' was found, or anticipated, in complex, func-

99

tionally differentiated and co-operatively organized societies. The impetus behind the transformation from one to another, an impetus which underlies all history, is the simultaneous growth in the size and density of societies (Durkheim 1983: 56). Weber was less concerned with this kind of transformation as an isolated generality but he did continually posit a progression from 'tradition' and 'communal' bonds to the 'rational' and purposively 'associative' in such contexts as types of authority and organization (see e.g. Weber 1968: 48–9, 215–16). There was also a general impelling force behind the transition, that of increasing rationalization. Such a force is finally secured in the dominance of bureaucratic organisation which itself responds to what 'the capitalist market economy . . . demands' (see Weber 1968: 973–5).

For Marx's work the concern with capitalism was primal. From capitalism and its creation, he extracted a force of inexorable productive efficiency which accounted for the evolutionary development of societies, a development which predicates 'a perennial tendency to productive progress, arising out of rationality and intelligence in the context of the inclemency of nature' (Cohen 1978: 155). To an extent, this perception of development was based on the comparative study of societies but it was founded mainly in the Spencerian tenet that all the stages of progression were contained, and could only be understood adequately, in their fullest development – that is, within the perspective of bourgeois society as the summation of history so far (e.g. Marx 1973: 105–6). Such a stance combined comfortably with that comprehensive xenophobia that characterized European thought in the late nineteenth century. This enabled Marx to judge and find abjectly wanting not only the primitive and peasant community but also the once elevated civilizations of India and China (see e.g. Marx 1969: 93–4, 188). In short, all these ancestors of modern social thought 'conceived of the new world in contrast to "traditional society", and behind this "traditional society" they discerned a primitive or primeval society' (Kuper 1988: 4). For all of them, demiurgic forces of progression create and sustain the link between modern European identity and what this identity is thus negatively derived from.

It is history which is supposed to have accounted for such transformation and effected the displacement of mythic accounts of origin and progression. It was only through the courageous acceptance of an illimitable history that 'myth could be left behind' (Eliade 1963: 113). Myth enshrined 'archaic man's refusal to accept itself as a historical being' (Eliade 1965: 85). But Occidental history has itself been revealed as mythic, both in its arrogation of universal history and its specific constructions (see e.g. Bernal 1987; White 1973; Wolf 1982). Despite its encompassing claims, it is a history limited also by its mythic form – a causally sequenced flow of events from an established origin. This undermines the claim for history to match, much less displace, an Occidental mythology. In its own terms, history is unable to sustain standard Occidental accounts of the origin and progress of society (see Hodgen 1964: 481–4; Kuper 1988: 7). 'Evidence' has to be found elsewhere. There have been two sources. One is the archaeological record rendered in developmental stages through its equation with a sequenced ordering of recent and existent societies. We have no choice, says Goody, but to accept the 'dangers' of this source (Goody 1976: 3). The other source of evidence is an anthropology which, as Fabian shows, transforms separation between peoples in space into separation and gradation in time (Fabian 1983: 11–21). 'We make up a story to cover the facts we don't know or can't accept ' (Barnes 1990: 242).

THE PROGRESSION OF LAW

These stories of the progression of society are intimately tied to and even told in terms of the progression of law. As Kuper tells us, 'the study of primitive society was not generally regarded as a branch of natural history. Rather it was treated initially as a branch of legal studies' (Kuper 1988: 3). Primitive society itself was 'a fantasy . . . constructed by speculative lawyers in the late nineteenth century' (Kuper 1988: 8). (Perhaps the study of legal cases in their temporally organized accumulation provided modes adaptable to ideas of the progression of society.) Furthermore, 'the issues investigated – the development of marriage, the family, private property and the state – were conceived of as legal questions' (Kuper 1988: 3).

Maine is the most persistently influential of the lawyer–scholars. His key and most significant work was *Ancient Law* (Maine 1931). The precise brand of evolution which he espoused is difficult to discover. *Ancient Law* was published in early 1861, soon after *The Origin of Species*, but apparently owes nothing to it (Stein 1980: 88 n. 24). Stein notes Maine's credo that history 'must teach that which every other science teaches – continuous sequence, inflexible order, and eternal law' (see Stein 1980: 88). He then draws a parallel between Maine's fleeting reference to geology and Lyell's 'uniformitarian doctrine' in which 'changes in the earth's surface were . . . the result of regular physical forces in constant, but gradual and almost imperceptible change' (Stein 1980: 88). (Stein draws a further parallel between this doctrine and the common law (Stein 1980: 88). Lyell was a lawyer as well as a geologist.) For Maine, regard ought to be had 'to the inherited qualities of the race, those qualities which each generation receives from its predecessors, and transmits but slightly altered to the generation which follows it' (Maine 1931: 96). There was an important aspect in which Maine was not like Lyell. Time and its effects tended for Lyell to be circular. He considered that 'the pterodactyle might flit again through umbrageous groves of tree-ferns' (see Gould 1987: 102). Advance, for Maine, was more resolutely linear, but it did have limits. After a certain stage, societies 'divided between stationary and progressive', the former having 'stopped' in their 'development' (Maine 1931: 18–19). Fortunately 'there were one or two races exempted by a marvellous fate from this calamity': they were able to form 'progressive societies' of which 'nothing is more remarkable than their extreme fewness' (Maine 1931: 18,64). In contemporary terms, the few were the advanced civilizations of 'western Europe' (Maine 1931: 18). Most famously, Maine discovered that:

> The movement of the progressive societies has been uniform in one respect. Through all its course it has been distinguished by the gradual dissolution of family dependency and the growth of individual obligation in its place. The individual is steadily substituted for the Family, as the unit of which civil laws take account . . . . [W]e may say that the movement of the progressive societies has hitherto been a movement *from Status to Contract*.
>
> (Maine 1931: 140–1 – his emphasis)

It is in such sweeping terms of movement from one state to its diametrical opposite that Maine sets the social evolution of the West. In legal terms, the achieved Austinian conception of law is radically contrasted to law's beginnings when 'it has scarcely reached the footing of custom: it is rather a habit': or, even worse, it is contrasted with a petty despotism in which man 'was practically controlled in all his actions by a regimen not of law but of caprice' (Maine 1931: 6–7, 152). In later work, first published in 1875, Maine tended more to what had by then become a standard notion of custom, one where custom is obeyed from 'an instinct almost as blind and unconscious as that which produces some of the movements of our bodies' (Maine 1897: 392). This was a scene in which the individual, and individual property, had little or no part. In all, 'Maine's theory of the "stages" of social development envisaged the march of the social unit from the primitive family group to the modern territorial state', his 'general thesis' being 'that the individual's power of self-determination increased even while the central political authority increased in power' (Stone 1966: 121, 126).

The mythic nature of this charter for Occidental authority is indicated by the oft-noted paucity of evidence Maine adduces to support it. Stein puts it kindly: 'It was Maine's apparently intuitive genius for generalisation that converted such ideas into the common currency of legal thought' (Stein 1980: 98). For the great bulk of Maine's story, the predominant source is Roman law, taken 'as a typical system' (Maine 1931: v). The supposed development of Roman law thence becomes a basis for condemning all societies but the progressive few. The lack of more extensive evidence was perhaps not of great concern to Maine since he adopted an evolutionary notion that secured his project in self-confirmation:

> If by any means we can determine the early forms of jural conceptions, they will be invaluable to us. These rudimentary ideas are to the jurist what the primary crusts of the earth are to the geologist. They contain, potentially, all the forms in which law has subsequently exhibited itself.
>
> (Maine 1931: 2)

Roman law provided both the simpler conceptions and their link to the progressive present:

> Much of the inquiry attempted could not have been prosecuted with the slightest hope of a useful result if there had not existed a body of law, like that of the Romans, bearing in its earliest portions the traces of the most remote antiquity and supplying from its later rules the staple of the civil institutions by which modern society is even now controlled.
>
> (Maine 1931: v)

Thus, Maine 'blazed a scientific trail into the fields of law' (Pospisil 1971: 150).

What would otherwise be astonishing claims for this strange little book – that it produced 'the common currency of legal thought', that its generalizations 'were then, and remain today, very persuasive' (Stein 1980: 98, 101) – manifestly have little to do with its scholarship but everything to do with its encapsulation of the myth of the age. *Ancient Law* was, as it were, written backwards. In an immediate sense, it implicitly addressed a debate on how India was to be governed (Stokes 1959). India was placed precariously in the progressive stream and could ultimately advance in the only way that advance could be made – like the Romans and the English. This revealed to the Occident a mythic progression that miraculously corresponded to its own self-presentation.

Accounts of law's progression by the originators of the science of society hardly improve on Maine's straitened story. Here, again, Spencer captures the ethos. His concern with law was frequent and I will take his chapter on 'Laws' from *Principles of Sociology* as the account which is perhaps the most coherent, if that is not to abuse the word (Spencer 1885: chapter XIV). This chapter is a miscellany of travellers' tales and occasional fragments of legal history. They are all held together simply by impelling verbs that, at best, evoke evolutionary doctrines. Thus, taking an almost random choice, the first few lines of page 527 reveal rules that 'grow up', laws that 'resulted from the growing complication of affairs', 'primitive sacred commands originating', 'a body of human laws' being 'produced' and one offence which 'becomes' distinct from another. The point of this catalogue, which could be readily derived from other parts of the chapter, is simply to show that Spencer had only to evoke what was by then the ubiquity of the idea of social evolution in order to establish its basic significance for law.

Of the three major ancestor figures of modern social thought, it is again Durkheim who is closest to Spencer. His sources are even more antique than Spencer's, yet he is hardly less confident in presenting a sweeping evolution of law which, in the opinion of later scholarship, succeeds in affirming precisely the opposite of what happened (see Lukes and Scull 1983: 10–15). The story of law, for Durkheim, is inseparable from that of the evolution of social solidarity. The origin of law is found in the emergence of organized sociality (Durkheim 1983: 34, 147). Law is 'that visible symbol' of social solidarity: 'we may be sure to find reflected in law all the essential varieties of social solidarity' (Durkheim 1983: 33–4). Conversely, social solidarity is 'in truth the soul of the law' (Durkheim 1983: 151). Law then, like social solidarity, is seen in terms of an evolution from one polar position to another. The origin of law is located in mechanical solidarity where, among 'the lower forms of society', it is penal, repressive and religious; its culmination is found in organic solidarity where law is based on co-operation among individuals, its sanctions are 'purely resti-tutory', its rules tend to be 'universalized' and rational, and where 'it is no longer wrath which governs repression, but . . . foresight' (Durkheim 1983: 38, 46, 55–6, 60).

Neither Marx nor Engels explored law in a sustained way but they were not inhibited in making the most expansive observation of law's evolution. Despite their devastating criticism of modern society and its law, these did represent the best in evolutionary attainment so far. Understandably, Marx and Engels placed par-ticular emphasis on the role of property and the development of productive forces in the progression of law. So, for them, 'civil law develops simultaneously with private property out of the disinteg-ration of the natural community' (see Cain and Hunt 1979: 53). But this kind of emphasis was not to the exclusion of other factors shared with the sociological mainstream, such as an 'increasing diversity of population', 'growing specialization of functions' and an increasing 'division of labour' (see Cain and Hunt 1979: 159–60). In the movement from primitive custom to law there was also a greater division of legal labour and a greater specialization of legal functions, and in this process law becomes, as Engels put it, an 'independent sphere . . . which, for all its general depend-ence on production and trade, has also a specific capacity for reacting upon these spheres' (see Cain and Hunt 1979: 55, 57). The evidence Marx and Engels drew on for their ideas of evolution was extensive but it was also diffuse and did not address the supposed evolution of law any more than sporadically, let alone match its encompassing range. Marx did not ease the demand for evidence by adding law to those categories, such as production and labour, which can only be fully understood from the perspective of their fullest development (Marx 1973: 105–6). It was Pashukanis who made the addition for him:

> The more highly developed form [of law] renders the prior
> stages, in which it appears only as an embryo, comprehensible

to us . . . . Only after a period of gradual development does it reach its full flowering, its maximum differentiation and definition.

(Pashukanis 1978: 70–1)

Weber, I suggested earlier, did not espouse an overarching evolutionary line but he did map out a progression in some particular social fields. These included law, the 'stages' of whose 'general development' he sketched somewhat in the tradition of Maine (see e.g. Weber 1954: 303). But Weber's persistent impact on conceptions of law is typified more by the processes of negation he used to identify modern law than by any comprehensive account of its evolution (see e.g. Unger 1976). Law develops in an increasing rationality and calculability (Weber 1954: 304, 350–1). These attributes, like other features of modern society, Weber extracts in a constant comparison with other times and places, especially the Orient, where such things do not exist. This is not a matter of superior Occidental virtue but of 'concrete political factors, which have only the remotest analogies elsewhere in the world' (Weber 1954: 304). Hence, there is a contrast between an individually based 'freedom of contract' combined with the modern territorial state and ascriptive membership of 'law communities' that are 'particularist' (Weber 1968: 695–9a). Or, in more operative terms:

Rational adjudication on the basis of rigorously formal legal concepts is to be contrasted with a type of adjudication which is guided primarily by sacred traditions without finding therein a clear basis for the decision of concrete cases.

(Weber 1954: 351)

'An abstract formalism of legal certainty' is constituted in the negation of the 'nonformal law' of patrimonial authority's arbitrary embrace or the Khadi's discretionary justice dispensed under a palm tree (Weber 1954: 351, 1968: 811). These travesties find modern equivalents in 'every form of "popular justice"' and 'every type of intensive influencing . . . by "public opinion"', both alike being incompatible with 'the rational course of justice' (Weber 1954: 356).

'It is merely in the light of our ignorance that all alien shapes take on the same hue' (Anderson 1974: 549). Even the uniform pall which these prophets of modern law visit on the negated world

106

cannot be recognized simply as different, for that would be to mark limits to the European project. Such difference is accommodated as a precursor to what inexorably and universally has come about. A whole world is appropriated in the constitution of European being. In its apotheosis, modern law moves definitively and distinctly beyond prior stages which are different to yet of it. The history of what modern law is not becomes also a history of what it is. This is the outcome of mythic dynamics that both propel the linear progression of law, and of society, and provide the standards whereby some are judged as having progressed less than others. These dynamics I have derived from ancestor figures of modern social thought but they have since become standard, their mythic content having been somewhat, but only somewhat, 'whitened'. Eurocentric, quasi-universal standards of sociality, of complexity or differentiation in society, of productive efficiency and rationality remain readily identified by the inadequacies they reveal in those who have been superseded. In its culmination, law is not only a product of these exemplary dynamics but becomes their instrument. All this is not simply a matter of theoretical perception. It was massively confirmed in the experience of colonialism.

COLONIALISM AND THE CONFIRMATION OF LAW

The amnesiac quality of modern law's origins avoids a momentous paradox. An advanced Occidental law, wedded in its apotheosis to freedom and a certain equality, becomes thoroughly despotic when shipped to the rest of the world in the formal colonizations from the late eighteenth to the early twentieth centuries. There were and had to be sufficient similarities between the metropolitan and the colonial laws to make them the same. Evolved Occidental law was a unitary, universal object. This law was a prime justification and instrument of imperialism, one which, in the assessments of the great practitioner–theorist of imperialism, would 'raise the mass of the people of Africa to a higher plane of civilization', a gift which should 'deserve the gratitude of the silent and ignorant millions' (Lugard 1965: 546–7). 'Our law', said Fitzjames Stephen about India, 'is in fact the sum and substance of what we have to teach them. It is, so to speak, the gospel of the English, and it is a compulsory gospel which admits of no dissent and no disobedience' (see Stokes 1959: 302). This legal tradition had been initiated long before in the colonization of Ireland (see Pawlisch 1985: 6, 14). The more immediate influence and the general modality of modern colonial rule came from the administrative formalization of the British rule of India and the impact on this of Bentham and other utilitarians (Stokes 1959).

The authoritarian and transformative character of law in the utilitarian rendition was perfectly suited to colonial rule. Even the more liberal of this tendency fell into line over India. John Stuart Mill, writing 'On Liberty', proclaimed that 'despotism is a legitimate mode of government in dealing with barbarians provided the end be their improvement' (Mill 1962: 136). The 'language of command', 'the instrument of law' and 'the immense and indefinite influence which the utilitarians allowed to the power of law and government' were to 'introduce . . . the essential parts of European civilization' (Stokes 1959: 55, 72, 302). Such a mission was also intimately tied to law in Europe (Gramsci 1957: 188). And, as in Europe, paradox is compounded in the claim of a civilizing law to bring order through the constant infliction of violence. Despite an abundance of contrary evidence, law was intrinsically and irrefutably associated by administrator and anthropologist alike with peace and order (see Faris 1973). Yet this same law was in the vanguard of what its own proponents saw as a 'belligerent civilization', bringing 'grim presents' with its penal regulation and, in the process, inflicting an immense violence (see Nandy 1983: 69; Stokes 1959: 209, 288). This contradiction was resolved in the mythic equation of order exclusively with an order that was imperially imposed. In mythology, as we saw in chapter 2, colonization is always associated with the bringing of order into a disordered situation. What existed apart from imperial order was the chaos of a pre-creation in which the natives lived, or barely lived, in anarchy, sorcery and terror. Any means of civilization is justified in dealing with this absolute and abject negation of it.

Despite the necessary similarity between the law of Europe and the law of the colonies, there was a large and telling difference between them. A legal order structured around the self-determining subject of Europe was, in its terms, the opposite of the authoritarian legal regime necessary for imperial modes of exploitation (Fitzpatrick 1983). This could not be a matter of a dissonance or deficiency 'in the path of the perfected law' which one colonial magistrate exhorted his charges to follow' (see Kelsey 1990: 212). The seeming diversity in law was resolved, rather, in terms of the character of these charges. 'The African', may have 'had a right to law' but not 'a right to self-determination . . . because the African had not yet found a self to determine' (Thornton 1965: 158). Westlake's *Chapters on the Principles of International Law*, published in 1894, found that:

> of uncivilized natives international law takes no account. This . . . does not mean that all rights are denied to such natives, but that the appreciation of their rights is left to the conscience of the state within whose recognized territorial sovereignty they are comprised . . . . Becoming subjects of the power which possesses the international title to the country in which they live, natives have on their governors more than the common claim of the governed, they have the claim of the ignorant and helpless on the enlightened and strong: and that claim is the more likely to receive justice, the freer is the position of the governors from insecurity and vexation.
>
> (Westlake 1971: 47, 50–1)

Such doctrines rendered the colonized as legal non-persons, able to 'enjoy the rights of man' only 'by means of European conquest' and then only in the dispensation of the European (see Kiernan 1972: 23). But as Knox recognized, in his critical vein, the imperial 'Saxon race' extended 'the rights of man' to 'no other races' (Knox 1862: 547). The good reason why can be illustrated in *R v. The Earl of Crewe* ex parte *Sekgome* (1910 2 KB 576). This English case involved a law of a British protectorate in southern Africa which provided specifically for the detention of a potentially restless native. An extremely enterprising counsel argued that, since this measure lacked universal application, it could not be valid law and the ancient remedy for wrongful detention, *habeas corpus*, would apply. The argument was rejected and the rejection bolstered in such sentiments as those best expressed by Farwell L.J.:

> The truth is that in countries inhabited by native tribes who largely outnumber the white population such acts [as the *Habeas Corpus* Act], although bulwarks of liberty in the United Kingdom, might, if applied there, well prove the death warrant of the whites.
>
> (at 615)

In such places the state's 'first duty is to secure the safety of the white population by whom it occupies the land' (at 615–16).

The European encompassed the very being of the colonized. Because of their higher position in the scale of progression, the colonists could know and represent the natives better than they could themselves. The most complex of resident legal cultures were taken over with an unquestioning confidence by colonial administrators whence they were incidentally but radically transformed. Even when legal regulation remained in local hands – an inevitability, given the limited penetration of imperial rule – they were subject to scrutiny and rejection under so-called repugnancy clauses in colonial legislation. With these clauses, local law or custom could not be effective if found to be 'repugnant to natural justice' or to 'the general principles of humanity' and such – criteria intrinsic, of course, to a universal imperial project. The potent implication of the repugnancy clause is that the native does not have a distinct and integral project since, with the repugnancy clause, a part of the resident culture can be denied here and a part there without any harm to a significant fabric of existence. Such an ultimate negation by imperialism was profoundly identified by Fanon as the fragmentation of a life once lived and the consequent rigidification of the fragments, the dynamic of which is now external to them (Fanon 1967). The colonized are relegated to a timeless past without a dynamic, to a 'stage' of progression from which they are at best remotely redeemable and only if they are brought into History by the active principle embodied in the European.

It was in the application of this principle that the European created the native and the native law and custom against which its own identity and law continued to be created. The small, static, kin-based group, bound by a barely explicit, almost instinctual and indolent custom, was created both in a fantastic inversion of European identity and by colonial regulation (Fitzpatrick 1984). Great civilizations were adjudged stagnant and fundamentally limited by the 'village community' which 'restrained the human mind within the smallest possible compass, making it the unresisting tool of superstition, enslaving it beneath traditional rules, depriving it of all grandeur and historical energies' (Marx 1969: 94). Histories of resistance to colonization, enterprises of pre-colonial history, of interpretative anthropology and cultural critique now evoke worlds of dynamic diversity, of protean identities, of labile and far-flung social relations and creative regulation, all of which imperialism reduces and arrests as in a mould – fixed, uniform and precisely contained (see Ranger 1983; Strathern 1985).

The shaping and control of native society involve another large and telling difference between the law of Europe and the law of the colonies. This is closely related to the difference I have just explored between a legal order involving the self-determining subject and a legal order where this subject is absent. In the colonial situation, law imports the same mythic forces it has in the metropolitan setting – universal potency, its domination of nature, its domination of lesser orders, and so on. But in this situation, law lacks the support of the detailed and tentacular non-legal controls that operate in the West and which go to create a self-determining, and self-regulating subject. Such a subject, as we shall see later in this chapter, does not make undue or destructive demands on liberal legality or on its pre-conditions of freedom and a certain equality. This self-determining subject was the antithesis of colonial rule. The detailed controls of this rule were provided by law, and law conferred on the colonial administrator powers of a range and discretion that would have exceeded the most expansive appetites of the Khadi or the patrimonial patriarch. This law made the whole of native society deviant, or always potentially deviant, never secure in any aspect from supervision, direction and correction (see e.g. Rogers 1987: 210–11 and Worger 1983: 51–2).

There are other ways besides colonialism and its effects in which the racial foundation of law's identity is set, even if these other ways are perhaps less explicit or more 'whitened'. I will consider two of the most significant of these ways in the rest of the chapter: first the nation and the nationality of law, then the modern subject and legal subjectivity.

THE NATIONALITY OF LAW

The mythic figure of the nation continues to sustain the force of imperialism. Not only did modern imperialism comprehensively extend the nation-state as a world model but the diversity of nations also maintains the distinctions of imperialism. Conversely, it is an imperialism, known by its proponents now in other terms, that inhabits and mediates between the universal claims of nation and its operative limitations. Nationalism imports a set of standards or norms which some countries, those of 'the West', are capable of attaining even if they are in various stages of so doing. 'The universal standard of progress' thus involved is 'not seen in any fundamental way as being alien to the national culture'

(Chatterjee 1986: 1–2). This capability is alien to other countries where it has, at best, yet to be proved. Nationalism, in the terms of its Western advocates, 'is coeval with the birth of universal history': it 'represents the attempt to actualize in political terms the universal urge for liberty and progress' (Chatterjee 1986: 2). As with imperialism, nationalism is an exemplary and expansive force, an infinite imposition on those who are yet to act, or to act fully, in accordance with its standards or yet to recognize them.

It is a common but still startling claim that nationalism is a product of the early nineteenth century (see e.g. Smith 1986: 11). Even the English, who claim exemption from such abrupt attributions, came at this time to exalt their nation and the civilization it offered above all others (see Curtin 1964: 143; and generally Newman 1988). Whilst the national identity of such 'old nations' as the English, the French and the Dutch long preceded the early nineteenth century, the claim to a distinct change at that time entails a purposive construction of the nation or the perception of its unique development, and the setting of it on a course which, if rarely specific in its outcome, was constant in its forward orientation. The vagueness of the destination did not inhibit an instrumental voracity of the nation – an open-ended subordination of life to the achievement of its indefinite purpose. The nation became the mode through which 'man' was now to make 'himself' (Kelley 1984a: 14–15). For Bagehot, in the English setting, 'nation-making' was the essence of evolution (see Hobsbawm 1990: 23). John Stuart Mill saw infinite benefit for the provincial in joining the British or French nation rather than continuing 'to sulk on his own rocks, the half-savage relic of past times, revolving in his own little mental orbit, without participation or interest in the general movement of the world' (see Hobsbawm 1990: 34). Where the project of nation-building was more explicit, as in Germany, the imperatives of subordination to a new collectivity tended to be expressed in more exalted and absolute terms (e.g. Strakosch 1967: 3–4). But wherever it appeared, the aim of achieving hegemony within the nation through the imposition of homogeneity in language, culture and law was tied to a universal progression in which the 'Great Powers' or the 'comity of nations' within Western Europe were at the forefront.

It was the mediating force of progression which reconciled this mythic elevation with the diversity and limits of more particular accounts of national origin and being – not that these were necessarily any more accurate than claims to the universal since, as Renan put it, 'getting its history wrong is part of being a nation' (see Hobsbawm 1990: 12). Whether recent and abrupt or immemorially regressive, national histories were constructed or reconstructed which, far from pursuing fraternal connections with other people in a universal project, told rather of exclusive origins and identity, of distinct community and a unique spirit. Present limits of these particular histories are transcended in their elevation as part of, or even as a prerogative purchase on, universal progression. The operative reality thus created – the fusion of particular identity and a universal project – has manifestly sustained an enormous existential commitment to the nation and generated a profound fidelity among its subjects, fidelity even unto death. No primitive or ancient mythmaker could achieve more.

Racism, as we have seen, inextricably occupies the ground of progression and here, in its relation to the nation, it assumes the role of the mythic mediator. Race gives specific identity to the nation in both of the nation's contradictory dimensions of the universal and the particular and, by 'itself' staying one and the same, it presents these two dimensions as likewise one and the same. Race gives content to particular nationalism by creating or, in a certain literal sense, embodying the integrity and purity of the nation. This is done predominantly by constituting the nation's identity in opposition to a racial identity which it is not. The 'purity' of the nation is a negative residue or reaction, the polyglot nature of which is unexaminable – it 'remains invisible' (Balibar 1990: 285). Its very intangibility allows of the most extreme and varied measures to protect it. Race, in its universal dimension, marked out a civilized 'Europe' and later 'the West' which, no matter what their internal diversity, shared an imperial comity over and against certain 'others'. The resulting identity in its arrogation of 'the general movement of the world' takes on a universal expanse. Racism is thus able to go between and unify the two dimensions of nationalism and yet remain the same, since it takes on an indefinite content in each location through a similar process of negation. 'True' nationalism, then, resides with the nations of the West. It sets norms of performance which other 'newer' nations can seek to achieve but to which they only, so far and in varying degrees, approximate. These norms exemplified by the West are transcendent and universal yet also specifically national. So, the use of 'objective' criteria, the achievement of a rational and 'industrial' culture, 'the establishment of an anonymous, impersonal society' (Gellner 1983: 57), institutional differentiation and the depersonalization of power are all values and achievements which can both typify the West yet be universal because of their ultimate constitution in the negation of what is local and personal, status-ridden, traditional, irrational, undifferentiated, agricultural, and so on.

Law's claims to universal, objective, impersonal (and so on) rule are made palpable and plausible through the mythic mediation of the nation. At first sight, the identification of modern law with the nation seems to be confining and contrary to universal rule. Modern law was explicitly set against natural law and the objective law of Enlightenment and their claims to a present universality. In the supposed Romantic reaction to Enlightenment, law was seen as informed by and dependent on the peculiar characteristics of each national community (Stone 1966: 88). The resulting fragmentation and isolation of law was heightened in the divisions between nations and in the self-elevation of particular nations to a superiority which integrally involved law. England had a long lead in this. There such 'juridical nationalism' was 'unique both in intensity and in durability' (Kelley 1984b: 25 – chapter XI).

Taking a conspectus of such peculiar virtue, we could begin with Fortescue's influential 'Praise of the Laws of England', published in the sixteenth century, which was given point in comparison with the deficiencies of the French (Kelley 1984b: 25 – chapter XI). For Sir John Davies, a leading lawyer and scourge of the Irish in the seventeenth century, English common law 'as the peculiar invention of this Nation' and as 'connaturall to the Nation' excelled all other laws (see Goodrich and Hachamovitch 1991: 159). Coke located mythic origins for English law in an ancient realm whence it emerged as paragon (Pocock 1967). Coke's towering significance for practical legal thought in the seventeenth century was more than matched by Blackstone's in the eighteenth with his ordering of the law 'in a spirit of nationalistic self-satisfaction' (Simpson 1987: 299). Dicey has been authoritatively hailed as the successor in significance to Blackstone for the nineteenth century (see Michener 1982: xvi–xvii). He consolidated and gave operative form to that conception of law which Austin provided and which has since dominated English legal thought. Austin's commanding sovereign, as the origin and foundation of law, was located by Dicey in a Parliament with limitless power. Such parliamentary sovereignty, Dicey claimed, was a matter of law but it seemed to have been his invention: 'the oracle spoke, and came to be accepted' (Simpson 1987: 378). The vacuity of Dicey's claim to locate the foundation of law and of the constitution has been exposed by Carty (1991). What is left is an assertion of national authority, an assertion of Englishness which, for Dicey, contrasted immeasurably with the deficiencies of the French and, especially, the Belgians. Inconvenient domestic entities which did not fit Dicey's scheme, like Scotland, were relegated in a blend of evasion and bluster (Dicey 1982: cvi, 24–5).

It is, however, a distortion of law as national to see its dynamic confined to the nation. The nation's law is one of the key components of a unifying nationalism. It takes on a mythic scale as the ultimate form of rule, as encompassing lesser and partial legal orders which it supplants or which become subordinate to it. But at first sight this universalizing thrust of law seems to be confined to the bounds of the nation. International law depends on the support of 'sovereign' nations. In standard terms it can only be a form of law that is incomplete because it lacks attributes of the nation's law, such as an effective mode of enforcement. Yet even if international law is but an extension of (Western) nations, it is nonetheless significant for being that. It is one of the means of legalizing the world – an imperial extraversion of Western nationalism as the carrier of universal norms. Even Savigny, that great proponent of the identity of law and nation (of law as the common life of the nation, as *Volksgeist*) was ultimately not opposed to a transnational systematic spirit infusing national law, especially when that spirit took the form of Roman law (Stone 1966: 93–4, 99).

Nor did the peculiarities of the English inhibit the massive export of their law or preclude an alternative tradition of connecting English law with other or wider systems (see Simpson 1987: chapter 12). Amid the great diversity of legal systems, Austin discerned 'common principles . . . to be found more or less nearly conceived' in all systems of 'positive law' – the savages were not included because, as we saw, for Austin they did not have positive law – 'from the rude conceptions of barbarians, to the exact conceptions of the Roman lawyers or of enlightened modern jurists'. However, 'General or Universal Jurisprudence' was only concerned with 'the maturer systems' of law and 'it is only the systems of two or three nations which deserve attention: – the writings of the Roman Jurists; the decisions of English Judges in modern times; the provisions of French and Prussian Codes as to arrangement', meaning as to their general organization. From these, in their capturing of the universal, 'the rest can be presumed' (Austin 1861–3: 350, 356–7 – I). Perhaps the supranational nationalism of law can be most dramatically seen in the two most significant post-Austinian attempts in jurisprudence to erect a pure or self-referring conception of law. Kelsen traced the legal existence of law to its validation in a founding rule, a *Grundnorm*. Here 'law' is ultimately and completely located in Western metaphysics, in a white mythology (Kelsen 1961). Hart's 'concept of law' has more diffuse origins, as we will see in chapter 6, but it does secure a primal foundation in a Western myth of progression which produces a Western positive law as the exclusive type of 'law' (Hart 1961). Even in analytical jurisprudence, there has been dissatisfaction with such quests for purity. Law is still distinct but now the product of a distinct cultural community. However, just to instance the most vaunted advocate of this line, law retains its more extensive dimension since it is still informed by the values of the Western polity, and such (Dworkin 1977, 1986).

If the workings of law in its distinct community are closely observed, what we find is not an avowed abrogation of law's universality, a recognition at last that it reflects the interest of a particular group or class or gender; we find, rather, law acting as an exemplary form through which mythic validity is given to unalloyed reality. There are, of course, continuing nationalist claims to the superiority of particular legal institutions but these are claims made in support of a universal virtue which is not so amply exemplified in less happy climes. The pronouncements of law characteristically measure and enforce reality itself. Recalcitrant actions and claims falling outside the domain of this reality can only be abnormal or insignificant. That which is outside is continually encountered and continually serves to affirm the rightness of that which is within. I have elsewhere illustrated this line of argument in a study of the legal treatment of racial 'others' in Britain, a study of legal proceedings as rituals of reassertion of a reality within which the suffering of these others cannot exist (Fitzpatrick 1987). This national yet universal reality gives effect to an operatively popular dimension of law. A nebulous popular spirit, seminally elevated by Savigny, expresses the popular in law, even if it is then subordinated to purposive legal modes, such as the very legislation which it was set against. So much is indicated by the analysis of Savigny in chapter 3. What an evolutive progression adds, through the medium of the nation, is the making of an involving, familial spirit into the custodian of universal reality.

The mythic mediation by the nation between law's particular and universal dimensions is, in turn, reciprocated by law. As we have just seen, law is itself a figure both of the nation and of that paradoxical supra-national nationalism. In giving effect to the national interest as a general interest, law subsumes particularity and in this same dynamic projects itself beyond the particular bounds of the nation. Although, as Anthony Smith notes, 'the legal aspect' varies in its significance for different nations, law is nonetheless central to the operation and often to the constitution of the nation: it erects and standardizes criteria of membership of the nation and of acceptable behaviour within it (Smith 1986: 134–8). Positive law, emptied of any necessary traditional content, was responsive to the imperatives of the nation-state, including those of its self-construction. And, as Austin confirmed, the very ability to make law was the mark and preserve of independent political society. A deep existential attachment to law is often claimed to be characteristic of the people of the nation (see Skillen 1977: 91). In all, it is hardly surprising that law becomes a potent figure of national identity or that it remains capable of representing the purity and integrity of a race which claims to correspond to, or encompass or protect the nation (see Gilroy 1987: chapter 3).

As for that supra-national or universal dimension of nationalism, law in Weberian terms is the very figure of the 'legal–rational' authority characteristic of modernity. And 'law' is now increasingly invoked with indicative facility as a universal measure of appropriate behaviour, as a new *jus gentium*. In her Bruges speech of 20 September 1989, the then British Prime Minister notoriously set Britain apart from the European project but nonetheless affirmed a common European commitment to 'the rule of law which marks out a civilized society from barbarism', and recollected a common heritage in which 'Europeans explored and colonised and – yes, without apology – civilized much of the world' (*Guardian* 21 September 1989). Those whose compliance with the rule of law, international law and such is needful are almost always of the Third World. Eastern Europe has recently emerged as an intermediate category and as a probationary member of the West, expected to progress rapidly towards full conformity with 'the rule of law'. The crowning affirmation of this sentiment was contained in the 'Paris Charter for a New Europe', adopted by Eastern and Western European countries, among others, in November 1990 (*Guardian* 22 November 1990).

SUBJECT AND SUBJECTION IN LAW

Two strands of my argument can now be brought together. One concerns the modern subject and legal subjectivity as mythic modes which, like the nation and the nationality of law, sustain that racial division creating law's identity. The other returns us to the beginning of this chapter and the question of how the individual could still be a foundation of modern mythology with the end of the transcendent, sovereign subject that bestrode much of the period of Enlightenment, and with the subordination of the individual to a reign of finitude. I will now deal with that question and in the process accommodate the sustaining of law's identity in racial division.

The sovereign subject was a primal being of such complete self-sufficiency that no explicit note had to be taken of it. As we saw in chapter 2, it was able to order the world and contain in itself 'the nexus of representation and being' (Foucault 1970: 311). The subject, in short, pre-existed and mythically impelled all knowing and acting on the world. Towards the end of the period of Enlightenment what happened, in one sense, is that this position of primacy is lost and an explicit, finite 'man' is born. This being is constituted by and within scientific and historical determinations. Man is bound within 'the human sciences' and 'the historical sovereignty of . . . European thought' (Foucault 1970: 344–5, 377).

> All these contents that his knowledge reveals to him as exterior to himself, and older than his own birth, anticipate him, overhang him with all their solidity, and traverse him as though he were merely an object of nature, a face doomed to be erased in the course of history.
>
> (Foucault 1970: 313)

Still, this man has assumed a difficult supremacy in some mythic existence beyond the trammels of the mundane and the temporal. This man is yet 'a source of order for the totality', is 'at the foundation of all positivities', and exercises 'sovereignty over existence' (Adorno and Horkheimer 1979: 9; Foucault 1970: 313, 344). The subject asserts a mythic force or impetus affecting a world in which it is included. This 'imperious designation' of the subject is 'ambiguous', man being 'a strange empirico-transcendental doublet' (Foucault 1970: 313, 318). The mythic designation of man in scientific and historical knowledge provides for man's capacity to transcend and master knowledge, including the knowledge of 'himself'. The subject is created or realized through growing self-discovery and self-mastery, a process mythically presented in varieties of progression. What the subject has yet to attain becomes the promise of fulfilment. There are no way-stations on this path of progression at which the subject's creative force can rest contented in some fixed achievement. The subject heroically transcends finitude through a present responsiveness that is without fixed limits. This responsiveness is not just in 'thought-conscious-of-itself' but extends to 'that *not-known* from which man is perpetually summoned towards self-knowledge' (Foucault 1970: 323–4 – his emphasis).

How can a present, transcendent responsiveness be operatively reconciled with the mundane finitude of the subject to which it is joined? In answering that question, I will 'use', as a focus and a foil, Foucault's search for the subject. To trace Foucault's ideas of the subject may be to follow an erratic, even contradictory course. But, quite apart from the revelatory nature of these ideas, the very contradictions between them serve, somewhat paradoxically, to locate an integral subjectivity uniting transcendent and finite dimensions. It is this subjectivity which provides a basis for modern law.

Foucault once saw the individual as a consequence of discourse – discourse being capable of creating and organizing its own objects (Foucault 1972: 40). But Foucault was never content with the mere attribution of a strange force to discourse and he came to see that he had been talking about power unawares. With characteristic provocation, he now saw the modern subject as a product of power and, more specifically, as a product of mundane techniques of administration. Power creates its own subject. 'The individual . . . is not the *vis-à-vis* of power; it is, I believe, one of its prime effects' (Foucault 1980: 98). Yet, seminally, for Foucault 'power comes from below'. It is not 'univocal'. Different powers occupy distinct spheres in 'disjunctions and contradictions' (Foucault 1979a: 27, 1981: 91–4). It should follow that there are as many differentiated types of subject as there are powers (see Foucault 1977: 127). Legal power, for example, would produce a legal subject as its particular 'artifact' (Teubner 1989: 730). Indeed, Foucault pursued his histories of different spheres of power, his 'genealogies', 'without having to refer to a [singular] subject, whether it be transcendental in relation to the field of events or whether it chase its empty identity throughout history' (Foucault 1979b: 35).

But Foucault also made more extensive claims for the subject. From his specific histories of the penitentiary, the asylum, sexuality and so on, he extracted a modern form of disciplinary power and a concomitant subject. This was a thoroughly subjected subject, one created in subjection (Foucault 1980: 97, 1981: 60). There are obvious difficulties about extracting a general idea of the modern subject from a few histories of other things, particularly when those histories are concerned to dispense with a general idea of the subject. Foucault did make vague claims about the ubiquity of power, about powers configuring in 'hegemonic' dominations, about 'domination [being] . . . a general structure of power' (Foucault 1980: 118–19, 1981: 94, 1982: 226). But just what effect these claims were to have for the creation of a more expansive subject was never clear, although some general idea of the subject was at least implicit both in Foucault's optimistic advocacy of resistance to disciplinary power and in his utter pessimism about such resistance, a pessimism grounded in the inescapable pervasion of power within which we were all 'small captive shadows' (cf. Foucault 1979a: 200, 1980: 82–5, 1982: 211). But when Foucault came to jettison power as his cohering concern, he discovered that his goal had been 'to create a history of the different modes by which, in our culture, human beings are made subjects' (Foucault 1982: 208). Those modes came to include the ways in which individuals make themselves into subjects who act effectively on themselves and others (O'Farrell 1989: 113–30) – 'the forms and modalities of the relation to self by which the individual constitutes and recognizes himself *qua* subject' (Foucault 1987: 6). The individual was reinstated as 'the *vis-à-vis* of power', as an autonomous agent and the distinct starting point from which power flowed (Foucault 1982). I will now somewhat reverse that trajectory of Foucault's concern with the subject and extend the connection between disciplinary power and a self-sufficient subjectivity.

Foucault's specific histories uncover the lowly origins and the contingency of grand and cherished institutions and ideas, including the idea of the individual subject as the centre of the social universe, as the yardstick of moral and political evaluation (see Minson 1985: chapter 2). The modern subject, as the individual, is not the noble, complete realization of an innate striving, one freed from the restraining ignorance and prejudice of the past. The individual subject is, rather, the product of disciplinary administration. Modern liberal administration embodies a particular coupling of power and knowledge which creates a particular subjectivity. Whereas in the feudal period, the notable personage was conspicuously exceptional, modern liberal administration provides technologies which render everyone notable. So, each individual became:

> a case which at one and the same time constitutes an object for a branch of knowledge and a hold for a branch of power. The case is no longer, as in casuistry or jurisprudence, a set of circumstances defining an act and capable of modifying the application of a rule; it is the individual as he may be described, judged, measured, compared with others, in his very individuality; and it is also the individual who has to be trained or corrected, classified, normalized, excluded, etc.
>
> (Foucault 1979a: 191)

How can we link this contained individual as a case with the individual as self-constituting? The subject may well respond formatively to a diversity of local influences but its response is not simply immediate and localized. The subject is not, that is, constituted as a fragmented automaton. Through its integrating production as normal, sound character, the subject operates in a general dimension by taking these influences into itself and making them effective: 'individuals . . . are always in the position of simultaneously undergoing and exercising . . . power' (Foucault 1980: 98). The subject exists, as it were, outside of and orders the diversity of powers brought to bear on it. The greater the number and diversity of these powers, then perhaps the more varied and complex, the more specifically mediated, the more 'individual' is the response to them. My account here would accommodate only those normal subjects engaged in this self-subjection. The recalcitrant or the incapable have to be corrected or cured. At that point, the range of voluntary subjection has to end but the standards generated in correcting and curing provide guides to the normal.

Where can this transcendent yet bound subject come from? One answer is that the subject's transcendent responsive capacity is itself purposively generated by disciplinary power. Even in their diversity, each sphere of power Foucault accounted for contains techniques producing a similar subject. These techniques operate not so much by way of negative prohibition but, more characteristically, by way of positive, productive application. And it is in that application that the subject is produced. The more visibly spectacular, the more palpably normalizing elements of such power can be seen in the ranks, ordering, dressage, lines of observation and regularity and the linear operation of time embedded organizationally and architecturally in, for example, the prison, the factory, the asylum and schools. Race also serves as a visible point of application of disciplinary norms, one that intimately links with such other sites of control as the quality of a population, 'health' and 'the body', 'family, marriage, education, social hierarchization, and property' (Foucault 1981: 149). All these elements of disciplinary power are brought to bear on the human being as (potential) subject through modes of application that promote self-reflection and self-correction. Such modes, by way of inculcating self-responsibility, sever the link between the individual and formative social influences through the masks, the silences and solitary confinements of prisons, the production of introverted psychiatric knowledges, the asylum's repeated punishments terminated only on the inmates' acceptance of self-responsibility, social campaigns against masturbation oriented around self-control, the promotion of identity in racial terms, and so on. These modes of application are mediated through techniques of the most intimate and pervasive kind that rely on and imbue all and even our closest social relations. The power of the parent, the asylum governor and the social worker is often exercised in such techniques – in 'insidious leniencies, unavowable petty cruelties, small acts of cunning' (Foucault 1979a: 308). In all, these techniques are indefinite and infinitely adaptable in their ranging over and constituting the whole person, constituting the person's very 'soul'. The resulting 'man . . . is already in himself the effect of a subjection much more profound than himself' (Foucault 1979a: 30).

The subject is created, in short, in terms of a distinct individuality that is infinitely responsive and responsible. The subject is a self-responsible, necessarily reflective being with the autonomy needed for those attributes, a being who acts positively in the cause of its own normalization or self-realization as normal. The subject has to be enormously skilled in its own subjection, in organizing and sustaining some stably operative unity among the multitudinous, divergent effects of the techniques that produce it. The subject cannot in all this be merely the inert effect of diverse techniques. The subject has to be free even if this is 'a culpable freedom', one attended with 'the stifling anguish of responsibility' (cf. Foucault 1967: 182, 247).

It may be espousing an old-fashioned notion, but with this reintroduction of a transcendent subject into an area that was to be freed of it, we seem to be left with the prospect of 'a constitutive contradiction' (cf. Spivak 1988: 274; and see Foucault 1988: 134). The diversity of constituting techniques or even the diversity of powers coming 'from below', no matter how similarly oriented, provide no guarantee of a unified subjectivity, of that supervening ordered and ordering subject that seemed to be required to make the particular techniques or powers effective and mutually coherent. On the evidence of diversity, we could more readily posit, along with many others, a fragmentation typical of modern subjectivity. Where else can this transcendent subject be found?

There is work in the tradition of Foucault which would more explicitly locate the modern subject in a general dimension: Donzelot's account of the creation in France of the modern family (Donzelot 1980). Minson helpfully draws parallels between Donzelot's work and that of Strakosch on 'state absolutism and the rule of law' in Austria (Minson 1985: 181; Strakosch 1967). The combined story is one of the formation of a private sphere and of the public/private division in the transition from the feudal to the modern period. The increasing centralization of the absolutist state bureaucracies and the decline of the estates was accompanied by a centralization of legal power and the elimination of the multitude of legalities – of the extensive, detailed and various controls characteristic of feudal regulation. These were not or could not be replicated within this centralized power and within its forms and modes of law. There was new coupling of power which, in a sense, replaced 'the old loose condominium of Monarch and Estates' (Minson 1985: 90): a coupling of the public domain of this centralized authority and the private one distinct from it. The private is the realm of the modern family and the modern individual. This realm is not impervious to the demands of disciplinary administration. Such demands are there accepted 'voluntarily' as an impetus and basis for self-regulation. For the private realm to operate in this way, a certain enduring distinctness and integrity, a certain independent capability, are necessarily involved in its relation to public power. So, to take Donzelot's concern with the family:

> It could even be said that this familial mechanism is effective only to the extent that the family does not reproduce the established order, to the extent that its juridical rigidity or the imposition of state norms do not freeze the aspirations it entertains.

> (Donzelot 1980: 94)

This coupling of power can be refined in its relation to the subject through Foucault's sketches of a type of governing or of governing mentality – governmentality, as he called it – which became effective early in the modern period (see especially Foucault 1979c). He set this in opposition to an authority and order which it displaced and in which the law was ultimately significant, the law of God or of the earthly sovereign. In the modern period there is now a predominance of 'new methods of power whose operation is not ensured by right but by technique, not by law but by normalization, not by punishment but by control' (Foucault 1981: 89). Governmentality is concerned with the ordering, the management of whole populations. But 'the managing of a population does not apply only to the collective mass of phenomena, or at the level of its aggregative effects, it also implies the management of the population in its depths and its details' (Foucault 1979c: 19). And this comprehensive management of 'life' can extend downwards, as it were, extend as far as the apt type or types of subjectivity and so join with that similarly effective power constituting the individual and coming in the plenitude of its detail 'from below' (cf. Foucault 1981: 99–100). Modern power becomes capable of 'an individualizing [and an] exhaustive analysis of the social body' (Foucault 1980: 151). And Foucault did recognize that what was involved in the transition to modernity was a general change in individuality. Disciplinary power accompanied that 'historical reversal of the procedures of individualization' which I touched on earlier where the exclusive individualization of the feudal period is replaced by a universal individualization in which everyone is rendered notable (Foucault 1979a: 191–3). The feudal power which 'consisted in relations between juridical

124

subjects insofar as they were engaged in juridical relations by birth, status, or personal engagements' gives way to a situation where 'the government begins to deal with individuals, not only according to their juridical status but as men, as working, trading, living beings' (Foucault 1988: 156).

The argument derived from Donzelot and governmentality could be summarized by saying, with Foucault, that for 'modern rationality' there is an integral relation between 'the reinforcement of . . . the political totality' and 'increasing individualization' (Foucault 1988: 161–2). This outcome is supplemented in that mythology narrated by Maine and others. The individual comes to be increasingly self-determining, breaking away from the constraining bonds of a natural community typified by those existent peoples who have advanced little or not at all on the scale of progression. The power and liberty of the individual increases in tandem with the growth of a centralized, rational political authority. The extension of individual legal rights is combined with a rapid spread of the governmental control of life – things uneasily reconciled in notions of participatory citizenship (see Barron 1990).

Marx piercingly saw through that scheme of things. In the transition to a capitalist society, that vacuum created in the demise of 'natural community' is filled by general economic relations which dominate the political power of a centrally organized nation-state. The 'dissolution of traditional entities places individuals alongside each other as independent, private persons whose special links take mainly legal forms' (Jakubowski 1976: 95). Law also encompasses and mediates between the individual and the now general social relations made possible by, to borrow a synopsis, 'the prevalence of money capital, by the commodification of labour and by the transformability of the one into the other' (Giddens 1981: 121). The individuality and the generality are integral:

> Only in the eighteenth century, in 'civil society', do the various forms of social connectedness confront the individual as a mere means towards his private purposes, as external necessity. But the epoch which produces this standpoint, that of the isolated individual, is also precisely that of the hitherto most developed social (from this standpoint, general) relations.
>
> (Marx 1973: 106)

This is a primal individual, the individual 'as posited by nature', the 'starting point of history' (Marx 1973: 346). But this new individual was an abstract being, a void into which social determinations poured:

> In bourgeois society, the worker e.g. stands there purely without objectivity, subjectively; but the thing which *stands opposite* him has now become the *true community* . . . which he tries to make a meal of, and which makes a meal of him.
>
> (Marx 1973: 496 – his emphasis)

The conjunction and the disjunction of the individual and the social totality have, of course, revealingly plagued liberal political theory in its efforts to maintain the self-sufficiency and dominance of individual being. One line of resolution is traced to Hobbes. There, as we saw, an encompassing individuality devours all its lesser manifestations. For society to exist the enormity of the individual's power derived from the savage state of nature has to be comprehensively subordinated to 'that great LEVIATHIAN . . . in which the sovereignty is an artificial soul, as giving life and motion to the whole body' (Hobbes 1952: 47 – Introduction). In the other line of resolution the individual retains a more immediate transcendence. Unger posits for liberal society an absolute prevalence of the individual, of 'persons who transcend the groups to which they belong', who have in its fullest 'that power to transcend the forms of one's existence which is a defining feature of humanity'. This power enables them to move beyond the stifling constraints of 'tribal society' and 'traditional society' where 'there is little sense of individuality as a manifestation of a universal humanity that transcends every particular role or status' (Unger 1976: 149, 154–5, 226). In a more modern yet more Hobbesian vein, Unger also sees 'the guarantee of social and psychological stability under liberalism' as consisting in the subordination of the individual, of 'his desires', to 'his' social roles:

> This social image of the self steps into the vacuum created by the chaos of the passions. It gives the individual an illusion of coherent personality in exchange for his submission to the demands of the group. Among these demands is the need to strive for mastery of the skills required for the performance of his roles. In this manner, each individual's supreme interest in the image of self becomes the linchpin of social

order; he is led, indeed forced, by that interest to keep the savage passions at bay.

(Unger 1976: 146)

We will, in sum, not be oppressed by society's dictates and our individuality compromised as long as we hold ourselves ever responsive to these dictates and 'voluntarily' take them into ourselves, making them our own. This is a Rousseauesque freedom through voluntary submission. For Foucault, subjectification is produced by subjection (Foucault 1981: 60). The subject in all this is not simply the passive recipient of floods of social determination. If the transcendent subject is to be subjected in itself, it has to match the range of social influences brought to bear on it and it has to apply the particular aptitudes making these influences operative. I shall now look at these tasks and relate them to law and legal subjectivity.

How are we to locate the specific self-governing capacity of the subject including its comprehensive responsiveness to society, the totality and such? It is here that techniques for the making of the subject or disciplinary powers clearly come into their own. But they are not alone, although it is difficult to hold ourselves apart from their forming influences and to gauge the extent of their company. The pre-modern influences of a past from which the fully-found subject is now liberated are bound to be especially opaque. Elias, for one, traces a 'civilizing process' in Europe from the thirteenth century in which norms regulating personal behaviour, such as bodily functions, are increasingly elaborated and refined so as to create and heighten self-consciousness and the element of calculation and, thence, self-restraint (Elias 1978). Foucault directs us to instances derived from Christianity. He saw the sacrament of penance as an 'incitement to discourse', an incitement to making sexual desire explicit, detailed and subject to account in a 'nearly infinite task of telling' (Foucault 1981: 18–21). Confession was always the pending focus for the examination of the conscience, for the sustained evaluation of one's thought and behaviour in the light of unattainable standards. These could be the exemplary patterns provided by Christ and the saints or impossibilist prescriptions of purity in thought and deed, compliance with which could never be assuredly estimated. The Christian had to be constantly aware, constantly on guard against the seductions of evil: 'Brethren, be sober, be vigilant, for your Adversary, the

127

Devil, as a roaring lion, walketh about seeking whom he may devour; whom resist, steadfast in the faith' (Compline). Such requirements were refined beyond the institutional bounds of confession, extending as they did to a Protestant self-scrutiny and self-evaluation. The proto-disciplinary gaze of a demanding deity also provided a check on adequate performance. All of which provoked and required a degree of self-awareness that must have gone a long way towards constituting that uniqueness, that singularity of each of its adherents that characterizes Christian belief. In this belief, the individual is transcendent over society or community, having free-will but also the responsibility, 'with fear and trembling' (*Philippians* 2: 12), for his or her own salvation. 'Men were thought of as "free" so that they could become *guilty*' (Nietzsche 1968: 53 – his emphasis). The responsible and the aware self is, in conventional Christianity, the adequate and complete focus of spiritual concern. This impoverished self is clearly not distant from its fellows in the realms of discipline, civilization and so on.

A similar connection is made by Foucault between the pastoral power of the Christian Church and those forms of modern power and of 'governmentality' we touched on earlier. This pastoral power, concerned with the whole being of individuals, was once 'linked to a defined religious institution [but] suddenly spread out into the whole social body' (Foucault 1982: 215; cf. Hill 1955: 16–17, 1969: 112). The Calvinism of the sixteenth century could perhaps be taken as a refined pastoral prelude to the ministrations of governmentality and modern forms of disciplinary power. Its primary concern was to foster a pervasive 'discipline' – the nerves of religion, in Calvin's terms – 'attentive to all the *minutiae* of conduct': 'having overthrown monasticism, its aim was to turn the secular world into a gigantic monastery' (Tawney 1926: 115). 'It was in that spirit that [Calvin] made Geneva a city of glass in which every household lived its life under the supervision of a spiritual police' (Tawney 1926: 117).

Law provides ways of generating a disciplined, self-responsible subjectivity. These ways tend to be deflected from Foucault's work through his conception of law as 'juridical', that is, as extending no further than transgression, judgment and punishment (Foucault 1967: 267). Foucault was concerned to contrast the power of those techniques intimately creating subjectivity with a supposedly antique form of power characterized by law. As such, law is typified by the occasional, discontinuous and repressive intervention of the sovereign from outside the subject, as it were. This is most vividly marked by gruesome exemplary punishments (e.g. Foucault: 1979a: 3–14). But even in this diminished conception, law provided guidance, often spectacular guidance, to be internalized and followed. It may in ways be fanciful, but there is probably much to Nietzsche's arguments that the old, brutal punishments, as part of 'the long story of the origin or genesis of responsibility', did not so much orient people towards numbed submission as render them supposedly autonomous and responsible (Nietzsche 1956: 190 – Second Essay Part II and see also Part III).

With the strategies of the criminal law in eighteenth-century England, Hay tells us, submission was certainly the purpose but it was effected by generating an active consent through the legal process (Hay 1975). Repressive power can be productive (Minson 1985: 44). Neither is law simply repressive. In the modern period there is a seeming increase in the resort to law as facilitative, to the involving ability of the subject to act creatively through law, so much so that the contract is often seen as the typical form of modern law (see e.g. Pashukanis 1978; and compare Foucault 1979a: 194). The operation of this facilitative mode obviously evokes and relies on a sustained self-responsibility. But quite apart from the facilitative, law does not operate only by way of occasional intervention responding to transgression of the sovereign's prohibitions. For Foucault law operated in this 'juridical' sense because law serves to present power as a negative restraint on otherwise free individuals, thus masking the operation of a disciplinary power that positively creates subjects (Foucault 1980: 104, 1981: 86, 144). But law also operates in less confined ways, providing detailed imperatives and quotidian guidance that resembles nothing more than power's all-pervasive penetration in Foucault's idea of it. Indeed, Hunt locates parallels between this idea and Gramsci's notion of 'the educative role of law' (Hunt 1990: 315–16). And E. P. Thompson's delightfully intemperate historic search for law tended to find it everywhere, inhabiting a great diversity of social forms including 'the definition of self-identity' (Thompson 1978: 288), a location which I explore later.

The generation of a self-governing capacity through these techniques and traditions still leaves large contradictions at the core of self-responsible subjectivity. How can an infinity of capacities and responsibility be accommodated in finite being? The new subject, the individual, is the centre of a social universe but its capacities for self- subjection – disciplinary, civilizing, religious, legal or any other – are ultimately private and voluntary. On what basis, then, can general or uniform social effects be produced through the subject? Not by persistent restrictions external to the subject that would restrain its transcendent potential – not, for example, by the old system of laws that supposedly regulated a world in which each person had a set place. Nor could there be persistent and positive restrictions within subjectivity: quite apart from the necessary failure of the philosophers or the scientists to find a basis for such restrictions, the subject had to remain free to respond to the infinite and infinitely changing demands of society or the totality. Yet the individual does act in accord with the mundane determinations and uniformities of social identity and this has to have some existence so as to be recognizable and applicable by the self-responsible subject. But this guidance, to summarize, could not definitively come from outside the subject, nor could it come from what the subject is. It came from what the subject is not.

In the quest for this negative being, we can return to evolutionary theory and its centring on the self-determining subject. Natural selection, as we saw, was premised on the adaptation and advance of the individual entity in the 'progress towards perfection' (Darwin 1970: 459). For man, this advance, whilst being an individual advance, was worked out and marked collectively in the hierarchic division of races. With the inculcation of popular racism in the second half of the nineteenth century, this fusion of particular being and racial identity became pervasive (see e.g. Mackenzie 1984). The subject stands in constant and essential difference to the 'native' and various other equivalents of the savage state. The native, despite some superficial diversity, takes on characteristics set in opposition to the self-determining, disciplined and distinctly individual subjects. So, a recent book on 'the future of law in a multicultural world' tells us, with an abundance of supporting citations, that:

In Africa's systems of political and social organization in which the stress is put on the group and its solidarity and in which all human relations are dominated by tribal and kinship considerations, the individual counts for very little. Not only could he not become the carrier of civic rights and responsibilities, but he could not emancipate himself mentally or physically from family and lineage ties.

(Bozeman 1971: 96–7)

Staying with 'the African', who tended to displace 'the Indian' as the Occident's main contrary, we have Lugard's supreme authority for the commonplace:

> In character and temperament the typical African . . . is a happy, thriftless, excitable person, lacking in self-control, discipline, and foresight, naturally courageous, and naturally courteous and polite, full of personal vanity, with little sense of veracity . . . . His thoughts are concentrated on the events and feelings of the moment, and he suffers little from apprehension for the future, or grief for the past . . . . He lacks power of organisation, and is conspicuously deficient in the management and control alike of men or of business. He loves the display of power, but fails to realize its responsibility. His most universal natural ability lies in eloquence and oratory. He is by no means lacking in industry, and will work hard with a less incentive than most races. He has the courage of the fighting animal – an instinct rather than a moral virtue. He is very prone to imitate anything new in dress or custom.

(Lugard 1965: 69–70)

Regulation among such beings could only be through the 'rigidity of custom' and be of a 'relatively automatic nature', a mechanical solidarity (see Haller 1975: 127). In all, the native would not be able to act on and determine its own being, to accept and sustain a project of self-definition. It would, hopefully, be otiose to relate Lugard's typical list to its counters in the identity of the Occidental subject. The precision with which they stand opposed to each other should suffice.

What is important, both for myth and discipline, is that these savage traits exist not only in opposition to but within the subject. The unevolved savage continues to reside in the civilized subject as a converse and provocation to a disciplined (self-) control. What is worse, or what is better for sustaining a constantly demanding discipline, savage ways remain, as Said put it, 'mysteriously attractive', particularly in their indulgence and excess (Said 1985: 57).

131

Man, in all 'his' nobility retains, in Darwin's judgement, 'the indelible stamp of his lowly origins' (Darwin 1948: 405). A reversion to or decline in the direction of that origin was for Darwin a possible prospect, even if he tended to be sanguine about the overall progress 'of the European and other superior races towards civilization' (Stepan 1982: 58). Thomas Huxley was more determinedly pre-Freudian, or post-Hobbesian, with his discovery that 'every child born into the world will still bring with him the instinct of unlimited self-assertion. He will have to learn the lesson of self-restraint and renunciation' (see Landau 1991: 58). The ultimate horror is that with the negative constitution of identity in Occidental myth there is nothing beyond 'self-restraint and renunciation' (Conrad 1960).

There are various other states supported by this myth which serve to constitute the subject in negation. Women and savages were often evaluated and made known in similar terms (see e.g. Carr 1984: 50; Freud n.d.: 145–6; Poliakov 1974: 273). Also, 'many of the ways of picturing the black and the working class were basically drawn from one interconnected set of ideas' (Jones 1980: 144). Criminality and poverty likewise could be drawn in terms of a feckless and instinct-driven savagery (e.g. Jones 1980: 146; Mosse 1978: 83). The equation of savagery and childhood was standard (see e.g. Lugard 1965: 70). Foucault's account of the modern invention of insanity, although often thought of now as overdrawn, remains especially revelatory on this score (Foucault 1967). The mad were constructed in terms that replicate savagery – impelled by passions, lack of control, animality, idleness, propensity to become even madder if given liberty, and so on. The mad were separated, denied a project, denied effective speech and effective being, denied any dialogue with reason, a reason which is confined to the normal and the calculable and which finds its existence in the full possession of one's self. Madness was 'a manifestation of non-being' (Foucault 1967: 115).

The elaboration of madness, the generalization of its negative standards throughout a normal population, fuses with the Occidental myth of identity in the most influential teachings of psychoanalysis. There were close parallels for Freud between pathology and savagery. The savage state was the domain of destructive instincts, untamed nature, hedonistic assertion and animality. It was disorganized and uninhibited: with 'primitive men ... thought passes directly into action' (Freud 1950: 161). The overcoming of these monsters in the child or the neurotic could be mapped onto the historical project of mankind. Both exercises share indistinguishably in mythic forces of progression and of culture ordering nature. These forces in the setting of Freudian psychoanalysis have their own fantastic myth of origin. The slaying of the father by his sons in the 'primal horde' and their entering then into a social compact create both the cultural community and its progressive impetus (Freud n.d.: 102–4). The resulting 'evolution of civilization' consists in the progressive control by positive mental forces of the attributes of savagery. This is the very 'struggle for life of the human species' since such control enables the species to survive and advance (Freud 1949: 2–3, 1985: 314). The judgements of Western ethnopsychology continue to find the unalloyed attributes of savagery in those who have failed to progress in civilization (see Collis 1966 and Manganyi 1985). But we are all savages now: the prey of 'dim mechanisms, faceless determinations' (Foucault 1970: 326), of unconscious savage impulsions which the subject does not know but which it could seek to discover and control.

All these negative exemplars of race, gender, mentality and so on import standards that are illimitable and inextinguishable. Not only could the subject never be sure of matching these standards, they could not in any practical or final sense be matched at all. Quite apart from their inherent indeterminacy, these standards are given contents, officially and scientifically, beyond the cognition of the subject. If the subject is infinitely responsible yet cannot assuredly know its responsibilities, constant apprehension and restraint are required on the subject's part. This operates positively as a constant impetus to fulfilment. The path to ultimate self-fulfilment is mapped in terms of progression. Rousseau foreshadowed many a use of 'progress' for the purpose of progressive subjection by subordinating his autonomous, free subjects to certain educative imperatives, since it is only 'at the end of civic time, when men have been denatured and transformed into citizens, [that] they will finally have civic knowledge and a general will, just as adults finally have the moral knowledge and the independence that they (necessarily) lacked as children' (Riley 1986: 248). The natured savage is the negative measure of progress, of how far 'we' have advanced beyond others.

The constitution of self-responsibility and identity in a negative mode is crucial, I suggest, to understanding what is otherwise a paradox in modern subjectivity. The subject acts imperiously on the world and is invested with immense power but is immensely restrained in its use through the subject's taking on the task of self-repression to the point of political passivity. How is it that for the necessarily reflective subject this enormous power is inverted, as it were, and contained in the creation, as Elias has it, of 'the individual as *homo clausus*, a little world in himself who ultimately exists quite independently of the great world outside' (Elias 1978: 249). This self-sufficient, this closed man, Elias adds, 'determines the image of man in general'; 'this kind of self-perception appears as obvious, a symptom of an internal human state, simply the normal, natural, and universal self-perception of all human beings' (Elias 1978: 249). Such a universal identity is gained and sustained in opposition to those less-than-whole entities and states that deviate from it. It is complete and complete in itself. It need only extend beyond its self-sufficiency for correction – for the restoration of that which it already is – and to observe in a settled self-congratulation that it is not as others are. The power of the subject need only be exercised in the maintenance of itself – in the maintenance of its subjection. 'The history of civilization is the history of the introversion of sacrifice' (Adorno and Horkheimer 1979: 55). And this is a necessarily hidden, unacknowledged sacrifice.

This powerful subject in its solitary transcendence has still to relate operatively to 'the great world outside', but it must relate to the world in ways that do not undermine its integrity. One such way is the mythic mediation provided by law. Law not only bridges the divide between the subject and the world but does so in ways that give effect to and maintain the subject's integrity and potency.

There is a certain persistent opposition between law and the subject. Once upon a time, so we are told, a person was bound by their position within an encompassing system of laws, whether human, natural or divine. A person's relations to all others were set within that system. But with modernity the subject is freed from such constraints. The subject is now outside of law but, in order to relate to other subjects, it now relies on positive law – a law purged of contents once inextricably shared with morality and tradition. With the consolidation of this law, 'there is no longer anything ontologically real behind the particular being' (Dumont 1965: 22). Yet, for the survival and operative existence of the subject, law as one of the 'various forms of social connectedness' cannot be entirely reduced to 'a mere means towards his private purposes' (cf. Marx 1973: 84). Short of the full perfection of order, whether obtained through Rousseau's education or otherwise, an omnicompetent rule of law deals with the interim shortfall of disagreements, deviations and imperfections. So, even in this narrowest relation to the modern subject, law must retain, as it were, something of a pre-eminence. In broader terms, law is commonly conceived as mediating between or 'balancing' an encompassing society and 'the transcendent value of the human person' (see Strakosch 1967: 221–2).

Where, then, does all this leave the autonomous subject? In a precarious position, as the unresolved antimony in legal theory between the dominance of law and the autonomy of the subject attests (Broekman 1986: 94). But this precariousness is attenuated by a mutual and mythically mediated dependence between the subject and law. By providing points of orientation in an otherwise labile world, law is obviously going to be at odds with the autonomy of the subject. Yet even if law can now do anything, it no longer does everything. As we saw, the advent of a secular, positive law marked a retreat of law and left a so-called private realm ruled by the subject as the self-responsible individual. This realm of freedom is constituted negatively. It is what law does not constrain. The subject returns the favour, as it were. The self-responsible individual sustains the integrity of positive law by mediating the disjunction between law in its transcendent, encompassing ability to do anything and law as particularly, actually limited. The figure of the individual, in its flexibility and intangibility and alterity (we are meant to act on ourselves), in its givenness, provides a mode accommodating the oppositions between these dimensions of law. The disruption that would otherwise flow from having the free individual as maverick occupying such a pivotal position is obviated through the individual's also being an effect of that diversity of power which creates the normal, self-responsible individual, responsive not only to the dictates of that power but to the multitudinous authority of law. In particular, the existence of this self-regulated subjectivity is a condition for the existence of modern, liberal legality. It was the absence of this subjectivity and its disciplinary supports that made liberal legality impossible in the colonial situation, as we saw. The integral values of that legality, values of the equality and freedom of subjects before the law, depend on this responsive, acceptant subjectivity. For example, the lack of freedom and equality inherent in the labour relation does not stand explicitly opposed to liberal legality because, through the subject's free and voluntary acceptance, it is embedded in the domain of the normal, of the unremarkable. The relation is a creation and a consequence of the subject's free action. It is hard to invest freedom with more irony but we could try with an example from Foucault: it is that same, acceptant subjectivity which mediates the divide where 'the general juridical form that guaranteed a system of rights that were egalitarian in principle was supported by those tiny, everyday, physical mechanisms, by all those systems of micro-power that are essentially non-egalitarian' (Foucault 1979a: 222). And, in particular, it is a subjectivity shaped by these detailed disciplinary powers that mediates the opposition between law and state administration, 'the antinomy between law and order' as Foucault has it (Foucault 1988: 162).

Law recognizes and makes its own this general subjectivity on which it depends and which it also affects. With the rule of law, the subject can only be involuntarily constrained through law. Law marks off an area of freedom and thus renders opaque the 'voluntary' self-subjection of this free subject through disciplinary power, economic power and so on. The subject recognized in law is the universal, autonomous individual – the given and ultimate being, 'posited by nature'. Sometimes lineaments of that individual are explicitly recognized in the legal protection of certain basic rights from legal and other intrusion. But this is a varying and uncertain protection. It remains subordinate to sovereign or constitutional legal processes and, more insidiously, it is subject to legal interpretation. The legal subject – the individual who is able to take action checking on legality, who is able to enter into and enforce legal relations – is constituted negatively, like the general subject of which it is a form. Being a child, a woman, a slave, being colonized or mentally incompetent, have all operated to mark what fully-fledged legal subjectivity is not (cf. Foucault 1979c: 16). The abstract legal subject is free and equal with all other legal subjects, liberated from all substantive ties and immune from all determinations not of itself. It could only be operatively constituted in terms of what it is not.

In its negative composition, the legal subject combines the histories of law and the individual. We have already seen that the mythic advance of law and of the individual were inseparable. The individual, like law, comes into increasing definition, into more explicit being, with the progression from a constraining, savage society to a rational, modern world of jural relations. I will consider Unger's *Law in Modern Society*, perhaps the most widely acclaimed recent work on the social theory of law, as an instance of how legal subjectivity is mythically sustained in the current scene (Unger 1976). I take this text as significant in its own influence and do not seek to achieve the impossibility of reconciling it with Unger's later work. Unger identifies three 'major sorts of law': one is customary law, another is bureaucratic or regulatory law and the third 'may be called the legal order or legal system' (1976: 47–54). Unger never says what constitutes the 'law' which all these 'sorts' share. The dynamic constituting law consists, rather, in a dominating concern with 'the legal order' and its taking identity in opposition to the other sorts of law. In almost exact echoes of Maine and Weber, the legal order is found to be a rare and delicate creature which 'appeared and survives only under very special circum-stance': 'indeed it may be impossible to find a single telling example of it outside the modern Western liberal state' – and such proves to be the case (Unger 1976: 52, 66).

Unger evokes a vague progression from one type of law to another. First an inarticulate custom, then a positive bureaucratic law and finally an autonomous and general legal order. This advance is matched, somewhat in the manner of Durkheim, with the progression of societies equivalent to each type of law. The story is quite standard if told sketchily. It is certainly no less fantastic and wanting in evidence than the tales told by Unger's illustrious predecessors. At one end of the progressive scale, a 'tribal', custom-based society is erected, one devoid of all the virtues to be marvellously discovered at the other end in Western liberal society and its legal order. Custom typifies a society of such an inert, mindless uniformity as to make its grimmest Hobbesian counterpart sparkle in the comparison: 'the mechanism by which the passions are stopped from wreaking havoc upon the estab-lished arrangements of society is an unthinking obedience to the official culture' (Unger 1976: 145). The 'normative order . . . may remain almost entirely below the threshold of explicit statement and conscious understanding' (Unger 1976: 62). There is an 'un-reflective consensus', and 'unreflective acceptance of . . . collective values' (Unger 1976: 103, 129). The 'reciprocities of custom' are simply 'tacit' and the tribal group's common 'view of the world' in its 'hold over the group is so strong that it need never be spelled out' (1976: 129, 142). The savage remains notoriously and conveniently inarticulate. From its fastness, this impoverished group divides the world 'between insiders and strangers', between a communal solidarity and 'suspicious hostility' (Unger 1976: 140, 143–4). This old Occidental reverie culminates in the discovery that this situation 'parallels in the realm of culture the pre-determined course of instinct in the prehuman animal world' (1976: 93 – see also 132–3). In this realm of eternal fixity, it is understandably 'difficult to account for . . . change' (1976: 263). Indeed change must be 'alien' for a people without any 'conception of the right or the good as something towering above the natural and the social world that surrounds them' (Unger 1976: 143). This leaves the rather obvious conundrum of how society could ever have progressed from such an inert state. The most favoured solution had been that some could change and some could not, or not very much, and the division was made in racial terms. Being a liberal and an avowedly critical scholar, this solution is not available to Unger so the conundrum is a 'dark riddle' (1976: 154). It is abruptly solved by Unger's 'postulating' in flat contradiction 'that in any society that can be characterized as human there is always a potential rift between ideal and actuality' and this presumably allows different states to be conceived of (1976: 155).

The chasm between all this and any ever ascertained or ascertainable condition becomes irrelevant when we realize that the whole exercise is oriented towards the identification of liberal society and its pristine legal order. Liberal society 'stands at the opposite pole from the tribal' (Unger 1976: 143). There is a connecting progression between them via the kind of society typified by bureaucratic law. Apart from a vague 'frankly evolutionary' and 'speculative hypothesis', which is put very briefly, Unger claims not to advance 'any general reasons why one form of society turns into another' (1976: 154–5). Yet there are plentiful passing evocations of progression. In Unger's terms, one condition disintegrates or shatters or passes into another which emerges with greater differentiation, specialization, division of labour and hierarchy (1976: 61–3, 103). And in a strange retrospection of 'interests' some few historical reasons are given for the final advance to liberal society (1976: 70). In the end, liberal society and legal order are created out of the deficiencies of prior societies – out of what is 'failed', 'absent', 'half-baked' or 'lacking' in them, some lacking more than others (1976: 100, 105, 110–27).

In the overall change from custom to legal order, an inert uniformity gives way to the vibrant and labile diversity of 'group pluralism', 'tacit particularistic standards' give way to autonomously distinct and generally applicable rules, and so on (Unger 1976: 52, 62, 66–7). This foundational and stark opposition disintegrates in contradiction. Varieties of tribalism endure:

> The distinction between strangers and insiders never wholly disappears under liberalism. It persists in the form of national, ethnic, and local attachments, and, above all, as a contrast between the public world of work and the private life of family and friendship.
>
> (Unger 1976: 144)

Furthermore:

> the degree of generality and autonomy characteristic of the actual operation of legal institutions in modern Western societies falls far short of what the prevailing political theories demand.
>
> (Unger 1976: 67)

So much so, that Unger finds 'the very assumptions of the rule of law ideal' – 'that the most significant sorts of power can be concentrated in government', and 'power can be effectively constrained by rules' – 'appear to be falsified by the reality of life in liberal society' (1976: 178–9, 181). His consolation is that the group pluralism which made the search for a rule of law necessary renders it impossible to achieve: 'men are condemned to pursue an objective they are forbidden to reach' (1976: 181). That characteristic bit of melodrama would seem to be saying that legal order can only be transcendent. The overall story is a mythological narration of its origin and progression.

It is the mythic figure of the individual which bears the burden of contradiction and irresolution in Unger's text. This individual emerges as the negation of the world of custom where 'each person sees himself as a barely differentiated part of a larger natural and social whole', where 'group standards . . . override and suppress independent individuality' (Unger 1976: 59, 130). It is the figure of the individual in its 'radical separateness' which can give meaning to 'social relations' rather than be given meaning by them in a tribal existence where 'order in society presupposes and evokes order in the soul' (1976: 57, 130, 145). Individuals can know and encompass diversity. They are the focal point of co-hesion for liberal pluralism since they are 'persons who transcend the groups to which they belong' – transcend 'national, ethnic and local attachments . . . family and friendship' (1976: 144, 149).

Following on but departing now from Unger, I should indicate finally how the infinitely mediative individual exists operatively and finitely in law. The legal subject shares with the general subject those negatively determined attributes of infinitely competent responsibility and self-cohering discipline, together with the autonomy necessary for those attributes. The legal subject draws together and indistinguishably absorbs the diversity of existence that is being in law. It brings to bear on itself and makes operative through itself the vast domain of guiding legal knowledge. The performance of the legal subject cannot be limited in terms of specific abilities or in terms of a specific awareness: ignorance of the law, for example, is no excuse. This negatively constituted responsibility is a pure responsibility, one which can be made to bear on anything at any time. It is a responsibility that extends to a limitless possibility of imperatives. The legal subject is bound not just to a law that most often cannot be assuredly known but also to anything the law becomes. As with general subjectivity, the legal subject is necessarily apprehensive and restrained in the face of that which is dangerous but inadequately known. This purely hyper-responsible subject could be seen as a not too distant cousin of the authority-ridden subject invoked by legal positivists, a sub-ject intrinsically obedient to law or intrinsically committed to it. This responsibility entails a mode of being that is inextricably attached to law (Goodrich 1990: chapter 8), one where there has been a thorough 'internalization of the juridical instance' (cf. Foucault 1967: 267). That attachment is also specific to law. As progression, as always becoming something else, law cannot simply derive operative subjectivities from elsewhere. It demands a specific allegiance.

In modern law, the subject is ultimately confined in terms similar to those that go to make the subject in general. The rampant will of self-legislating subjectivity is reduced to the lonely will of *homo clausus*, separated from and set against all others. For von Jhering, 'the progress of law consists in the destruction of every natural tie, in a continued process of separation and isola-tion' (see Diamond 1973: 326). And for Pashukanis, 'the juridical element in the regulation of human conduct enters where the isolation and opposition of interests begins' (Arthur 1978: 13). In its isolation, in its solitary subjection, the legal subject has to be organized purely internally. It cannot, as it were, stand on some external base and range securely from there. The legal subject is continually and apprehensively engaged in erecting, policing and adapting its own limits. To cohere and yet relate to others, the subject 'must have become not only calculating but himself calculable, regular even to his own perception, if he is to stand a pledge for his own future as a guarantor does' (Nietzsche 1956: 190 – Second Essay, I). The basis on which the legal subject relates to others is ultimately a contract with the self which is also a self-contraction – *homo contractus* perhaps. A mythic fate is avoided by ensuring it is not confronted. For Renner, the Code Napoléon 'fundamentally proclaimed only two commandments: a material one, that everyone should keep what he had, and a personal one, that everyone should mind his own business' (see Tigar and Levy 1977: 256).

By way of summarizing my concern with legal subjectivity, this straitened and withdrawn subject we have just encountered could be seen as the exact opposite of the sovereign subject which went out naming and ordering the world. Instead of constituting and dividing the world in difference, the new subject occupies a con-signed realm within an encompassing progression towards the realization of the whole. But this very progression is impelled by and creates a differentiation in which some entities assume an evolved, exemplary position. The entity as exemplar progresses and accumulates identity in the negation of antithetical, inadequate forms that preceded it. The new subject and modern law are both created in this way. They take identity in a mode which identifies them with each other. The division between the rule of law and the autonomous subject is mythically overcome. Race and nation, as we saw, provide participatory forms of that identity – in both senses.

PROGRESS AND ORDER IN LAW

That leaves a problem of how law in a world of pervasive change and progression can be reconciled with a law that persists as order. The lineaments of this conflict and of its resolution emerged in the consolidation of a modern idea of law towards the end of the nineteenth century. This was a consolidation around Austin's *The*

Province of Jurisprudence Determined (1861–3). One of the consolid-
ators noted in 1880 that 'there have been of late years signs of a
change in the mental habit of English lawyers' due mainly to the
influence of Austin to whom 'most Englishmen are indebted for
such ideas as they possess of legal methods'; Austin had put
matters now 'in so clear a light that they can hardly again be lost
sight of' (Holland 1924: vi–vii). This is from Holland's *The Elements
of Jurisprudence*, for long the most widely used text on the subject.
In its archetypal blandness this work saved law from Austin's more
extensive concerns. There was a:

> turning inward upon law and [a] losing [of] the vital and
> continuing inspiration for it which came from the deter-
> mination to understand legal phenomena on the basis of a
> general philosophy of the world in general and the fields of
> the social sciences within it. . . . It is symptomatic of what
> happened to Austin in the hands of his successors that
> Holland treats as digressions, spoiling Austin's systematic
> treatment of his subject, Austin's treatment of the psychology
> of the will, codification and utilitarianism.
>
> (Morison 1982: 151–2)

The purpose of Holland's text was 'to set forth and explain those
comparatively few and simple ideas which underlie the infinite
variety of legal rules' (Holland 1924: 1). One of the simplest of
these ideas confined law 'in the strict sense of the term' to
'positive' law of an Austinian kind, that is, law 'enforced by a
sovereign political authority' (Holland 1924: 43). This purification
or 'whitening' of law in its terms confined law to 'political society',
so leaving a trace of origin in the negation of the natural or savage
state by political society (Holland 1924: 47; cf. Austin 1861–3: 176,
184 – I). It is the narrow rendition of Austin that became, and
remains as I show in my last chapter, 'the staple of jurisprudence
in all our systems of legal education' (see Stein 1980: 86).

The ready reduction of Austinian law would, in its pure and
'scientific' ethos, seem to stand opposed to that other great contemporary pillar of jurisprudence, the historical school. The
leading figure in its English manifestation was Maine. We could
naïvely expect to find Maine pitting the irreducible richness and
diversity of history against the monadic simplicity of this Austinian
idea of law. In some ways Maine and others of the school were
disparaging of Austin, but one of the ways was that Austin had

142

taken too broad a range of matters into account in his jurisprudence (see Sugarman 1991: 46–7). For Maine, the Austinian idea was the culmination of law's progression: its components 'tally exactly with the facts of mature jurisprudence' and 'the farther we penetrate into the primitive history of thought, the farther we find ourselves from [this] conception of law' (Maine 1931: 6).

Here is an origin for that seemingly complementary division encountered in the first chapter between law as positive and autonomous and law as socially or historically contingent. As positive, law in its self-validating authority simply is. It affects its subject like a mythic fate. The exclusion of wider influence on jurisprudential ideas of law in the later nineteenth century is matched by the contemporaneous separation of a narrowly professional and singular form of law from other forms of regulation (Arthurs 1985). Law acquired purity and autonomy in both conception and practice. Outside elements are, of course, taken into law, but law does not cede their ultimate origin apart from its own self-regulation. It sets the terms of their acceptance and makes their existence dependent on change or abolition through legislation or some other purposive 'sovereign' process. On the other hand, law develops or changes with social and historical development or change. As it is so often put, law is responsive to 'changing social attitudes', and would cease to be viable if it were too long or too much 'out of step' with change in society.

I will begin the search for a mythic reconciliation of these contradictory positions and begin a summary of much of this chapter's arguments in what may seem at first a diversion. Sausurre introduced two senses of understanding into modernity when he located two 'viewpoints' in the study of linguistics, the synchronic and the diachronic. For him, 'the opposition between the two . . . is absolute and allows no compromise' (1966: 87). Both in linguistics and in the appropriation of these terms within the social sciences, the synchronic imports structure, fixity and atemporality, whereas the diachronic imports process, change and history. The distinction can be refined in something of its equivalent in linguistics, also introduced by Sausurre – the distinction between *langue* and *parole*. *Langue* is language as system, usually seen as rule-governed, abstract and unchanging. It is 'a self-contained whole' (Sausurre 1966: 6), having no specific connection with language use. *Parole* is the quotidian use and production of language. It is unstable, variable and socially determined. Lévi-Strauss saw myth as partaking of both *langue* and *parole* but also as 'an absolute entity on a third level . . . distinct from the other two' (1968: 210). He distinguishes between the two in terms of '*langue* belonging to a reversible time, *parole* being non-reversible' (1968: 209). Keeping these 'different time referents . . . in mind':

> we may notice that myth uses a third referent which combines the properties of the first two. On the one hand, a myth always refers to events alleged to have taken place long ago. But what gives the myth an operational value is that the specific pattern described is timeless; it explains the present and the past as well as the future.
>
> (Lévi-Strauss 1968: 209)

Myth, in short, 'overcomes the contradiction between historical, enacted time and a permanent constant' (Lévi-Strauss 1986: 16).

The myth of progression, which we have already encountered often, explicitly parades these characteristics of myth in general. The very progression from the primitive to the modern, from the simple to the complex, from the homogenous to the heterogeneous and so on, fundamentally involves an increasing differentiation in form and function. The story of progression comes in retrospect to be the story of a constant, enduring entity, developing in the negation of its origins and prior manifestations, always moving towards greater differentiation and autonomy. Myth revealed the 'full manifestation' of a thing (see Eliade 1968: 16). Even Marx's version, putting perhaps the greatest emphasis on historical determination, maintains the entity in some transcendent, 'simple' form (see e.g. Marx 1973: 105–6).

Law is created in a progression from the indistinguishable to the distinct. Again the point has been much illustrated already. To continue with strong cases, Pashukanis, in applying the evolutionist Marx to law, found that the:

> legal form persists for a long time in an embryonic state, with minimal internal differentiation, and with no clear demarcation from neighbouring spheres (mores, religion). Only after a period of gradual development does it reach its full flowering, its maximum differentiation and definition.
>
> (Pashukanis 1978: 71)

And it achieves this in the present, in bourgeois society. Savigny, the originator of the historical school, saw law developing to become the preserve no longer of the whole community but of specialist lawyers: it becomes more artificial and complex and a distinct science, although the popular element in law is preserved in the nebulous and indeterminate hold which the folk still have on it (Savigny 1831: 28–9).

To borrow a conclusion from Gurvitch, his account of the 'forerunners and founders' of the sociology of law shows that these ancestors tied law to the nation-state in a culmination of legal development that displaced or absorbed prior forms of law and custom. Such an outcome is extended, at least implicitly, in this scholarship to favour the claims of the 'inclusive' society over all 'included' social forms (Gurvitch 1947: 72– 96). The state-centred, formalistic 'prejudices of the dogmatic jurists' are thus upheld (Gurvitch 1947: 77). In myth, validity is conferred only on that which comes from the centre.

5

LAW AND MYTHS

There is nothing lacking compensation in something else.
(Borges 1970: 146)

THE MUTUALITY OF MYTHS

There is a certain mutuality to myths. They exist in a 'mythical field' (Lévi-Strauss 1987: 55). There a myth will depend on other myths for its 'full' meaning and effect. This is usually and accurately seen as a matter of supporting similarities between myths (e.g. Leach 1969: 22). But a myth self-evidently retains distinctness and difference from other myths. In this, a myth opposes other myths in the field. The mythical field, I argue, is one of mutual relations of opposition and support, of autonomy and dependence. The relation of mutual support and dependence becomes attuned to the cause of a myth's autonomy when that autonomy is challenged, either by an opposing myth or by a mundane reality. In those events, another myth will, as it were, compensate for the shortfall in autonomy exposed by myths or a resistant reality. We have already seen myths of law and of the individual relating to each other in this way.

In this chapter, I want to expand that argument in three concurrent perspectives. One simply presents the argument more explicitly and explores other myths in their integral relation to law. Another orients that exploration towards the basic jurisprudential divide outlined in chapter 1 between law as autonomous and law as dependent on society, providing reasons for what appeared there to be an inescapable coupling of these two types of law. With the third perspective, there is some resolution of persistent puzzles in the study of law, and the academic utility of seeing law as myth

146

is thus further established. These puzzles involve the supposed antinomies between law and two types of regulation. One type is heir to the objective natural law of Enlightenment and takes the mythic form of a scientific administration split off from a legal domain (see MacIntyre 1981: chapter 7; Arthurs 1985). In standard stories, with the advance of the regulated society, law is increasingly subordinate to an administration which it serves by becoming instrumental in purpose, discretionary in form and particularistic in application. The rule of law – as general in application, predictable and autonomous – is thus undermined. These qualities are also lost in another type of regulation displacing law: what Turk calls the 'return to primitivism' (1980: 16). Here the rule of law is opposed by substantive justice in particular communities. I will now consider these two derogations from law in turn, beginning with a challenge to the predominance of administration.

LAW IN THE ADMINISTERED WORLD

The revival of law in both Eastern and Western Europe challenges that strong intellectual and political tradition connecting law's decline with the advance of modern administration. There is also a persistence, even expansion, of administration along with this revival of law. Both the proponents of law's revival and the prophets of its demise would agree that administration and the rule of law are opposed. They would disagree over whether law is ultimately subordinate to administration or ultimately able to control it. This very disagreement points towards dimensions of the relation between law and administration which these positions overlook. If, with Foucault's considerable help, we identify a symbiotic link between the rule of law and modern administration, we then find that law is subordinate to administration yet also controls it. If we would resolve this paradox, we need to identify the limits of law and of administration in their relation to each other – limits which each is unable to reconcile with its own self-presentation as a general or transcendent mythic object.

The death of law is an over-heralded event. Unger (1976) provides a typical account. The story goes that 'legal order' or the rule of law was created in specific, even fragile conditions (Unger 1976: 66–86). As these conditions pass, so does legal order. In this mythic mode, an entity is identified by its origins. The possibility of other, supervening and sustaining, conditions is not considered.

In the coming of 'postliberal society' the rule of law is 'undermined' with the advent of a 'welfare state' and 'the overt intervention of government in areas previously regarded as beyond the proper reach of state action' (1976: 192–3). Formal and general prescription characteristic of the rule of law gives way before 'an escalating use of open-ended standards and a swing toward purposive legal reasoning' (1976: 195). The stock assumption is that changes in society somehow produce equivalent changes in law. A refinement would observe that law, in crudely quantitative terms, does not appear to decline but, on the contrary, to burgeon. With the growth in state welfare and regulation there is an increasing 'juridification'. But this juridification is at the expense of law's integrity or autonomy since law becomes more and more a conduit for the demands of administration (Teubner 1987).

There have been powerful claims of late in Western Europe that juridification is being reversed. Various combinations of 'neo-conservatism' and neo-liberalism provide programmes for reversing state intervention, resurrecting the market and reviving a classic rule of law. The practical effects have been significant and they have not been confined to places where such new or resurrected creeds are explicitly adopted. But these effects appear to be deeply ambiguous. Take the British situation as an instance. There the reversal of state intervention in some areas has been accompanied by its overall expansion and the state, more than ever, has attempted to inculcate a conformist discipline in its subjects (Fitzpatrick 1988a). The market itself has been vaunted not just as a liberation from state regulation, but as a means of introducing greater discipline, especially self-discipline, including an appreciation of the inevitability of authority and hierarchy. The very incoherence of such positions and the seeming inconsistency between neo-liberalism and neo-conservatism could be readily exploited (see Habermas 1990). The elevation of the rule of law could be set against the elevation of order and administration. But what I will explore is the ultimate coherence between such things, the mythic truth of their combination.

Intriguing parallels have now emerged in Eastern Europe. The *Paris Charter for a New Europe* adopted in November 1990 commits the countries of Eastern Europe to the rule of law, as we saw in the last chapter. But the situation also has its ambiguities in Eastern Europe. There the rule of law is supposedly adopted to counter state domination and to aid in a revival or creation of the market.

148

Although administration may not increase with the revival of law in this case, accounts of its decline are certainly exaggerated. Further, a certain reluctance about the market is more than matched by 'a similar reluctance when it comes to taking law and the rule of law seriously' (Sajo 1990: 329). Despite considerable disregard for the rule of law and the persistence of state domination, the rule of law has acquired effectiveness as a symbol of transformation in which 'the autonomy of civil (private) action presupposes a legally strictly bounded state: a kind of rule of law over the state' (Sajo 1990: 394).

What these two situations – a fusion of neo-liberalism and neo-conservatism in Western Europe and something of an equivalent in Eastern Europe – indicate is contrary to standard notions of the antinomy between the rule of law and administration. They suggest instead an operative compatibility between them. It is that compatibility which I now go on to locate and explore in the context of liberal society. I do this, first, by looking at the antinomy not so much in those well-rehearsed terms of the degradation of law but rather in terms of administration and how its pervasive and tentacular penetration inevitably displaces or, at least, marginalizes law. Yet this, I next argue, is only part of the story. If we consider the nature of modern administration itself, we find that it is bound by certain operative limits. It is in those very limits that the rule of law assumes a dynamic existence, one distinct from and opposing an administration to which it forms a necessary supplement. Moreover, in this relation to administration, law itself is limited by and dependent on administration. A contradiction is involved in which law and administration are integral yet necessarily opposed. Law and administration in their mythic mutuality limit each other yet sustain the claim of each to be unlimited. I will now deal with this compressed agenda.

Examinations of law's morbidity have tended to assume the inviolability of its causes. In these accounts, the welfare state or state administration or corporatism, causes the decline or death of law, or the loss of its autonomy or formal integrity. This process is seen as one of inexorable derogation from a prior and purer state of law when, as the rule of law, it operated with an independence and formal force which has since been lost or gravely diluted. This fall is traced to the domination of extensive state administration from the late nineteenth century onwards (see e.g. Dicey 1962; Hayek 1944). The direction of my argument is very different. It focuses primarily on administration rather than on law and it looks at the relation between them in that perspective. This enables us to locate these supposedly corrosive effects of administration right at the origin of modern law and to locate them as integral to it, rather than as something coming later and, as it were, from the outside.

I continue to draw on Foucault and his work on power for this perspective on administration and then focus it on law. This raises an initial problem. The history of France may not be the history of the world. Foucault's particular histories, such as those of the prison and the asylum, often make wide, implicit claims for their coverage and they have been criticized for this. My 'position' is that, in these more extensive claims, Foucault's stories may be too chronologically compressed but that, if we extend their temporal scope, they do provide a cogent account of profound changes in social regulation in the West. There is also his more general accounts of the emergence of a governing mentality, or 'govern-mentality' as he calls it. These are not confined to France.

Bentham should also be seen as a significant source here. For Foucault, Bentham gave analytical and operative form to a new kind of power within a new 'disciplinary society'. Such a power 'can be exercised continuously in the very foundations of society, in the subtlest possible way'. It 'functions outside of the sudden, violent, discontinuous forms that are bound up with the exercise of sovereignty' and are typified by law (Foucault 1979a: 208–9). This 'dispensing with the need for the prince' (Foucault 1979a: 208) does not go readily with the more English Bentham, with the modern begetter, via Hobbes, of an illimitable sovereignty given effect by law as its command or the expression of its will. Powerful as this law was, for Bentham it could also serve, in the more liberal strand of utilitarianism, to mark an area of freedom beyond its restraints. Yet that area of freedom was not immune to the new 'mechanisms of discipline . . . their spread throughout the whole social body' (Foucault 1979a: 209). With Bentham as the aspirant 'Newton of the moral sciences', any contradiction in this was overcome through truth and order being mutually dependent (Bentham 1970b: 273). Order like truth could be complete. The enfranchised could find their fullest being in a vision of total order, even if it was for Bentham a promised land yet to be reached (see Stokes 1959: 295). What can thus be found in the scheme of domestic imperialism initiated by Bentham, as I now hope to show, are the lineaments of a 'liberal' order and truth in which law and disciplinary administration are integrated yet maintained as distinct.

Foucault's concern with power was set against the figure of a unified 'Law-as-Sovereign' which occasionally and discontinuously intervenes in a society from outside or above it (Foucault 1981: 88-9, 97). 'In Western societies since the Middle Ages, the exercise of power has always been formulated in terms of law' (1981: 87). Foucault exhorts us to escape from this way of seeing power as superordinate prohibition or coercion – that which is subjected to power being otherwise free. Rather, 'power comes from below' and it does not leave vacant areas of freedom because 'power is everywhere' (1981: 93-4). We must find power in 'its real and effective practices', in 'direct and immediate relationships' with its object, in 'its material instance', 'in its ultimate destination' (1980: 96-7). This concern with power as operative was encapsulated by Foucault in terms of modalities – in terms of techniques, instruments, tactics, mechanisms – which operated in a dimension of the 'micro' and the intimate (e.g. 1980: 97-103). In short, what was distinctive of 'these new technologies of power' was 'their concrete and precise character, their grasp of a multiple and differentiated reality' and their ability in this to gain 'access to individuals themselves, to their bodies, their gestures and all their actions' (1980: 125, 151-2).

Power does not, however, simply meander among numberless instances. Foucault discerned a general change in the modern period from a type of power marked by centralized sovereignty and occasional or discontinuous interventions in society to a type of power that is disciplinary and continuously regulative and which pervasively, intimately and integrally inhabits society. It is a type of power and control not just, or so much, grounded in prohibition but more in the positive constitution of norms and the positive shaping of individuals to fit those norms. It is brought into effect within numerous particular fields of power dealing with, for example, crime and the prison, health, education, urban life, the control of mobility, recreation, morality, the workplace, the asylum, race and sexuality. Perhaps the most spectacular contrast Foucault provides is that between the conventional view of the negative repression, 'the refusal of recognition', of sexuality in systems of power in the West in the nineteenth century and the view in the first volume of his 'history of sexuality' which reveals the burgeoning of sexuality in this period as a field of public control and private self-regulation (Foucault 1981: 69). For the general presence of disciplinary power what is relevant is the intimidating, massively shaping effect of the interacting sum of these fields of power. Although disciplinary power latches most palpably and intentionally onto the abnormal and the deviant (Foucault 1979a: 193), it also has to be seen as a generalized effect operative throughout the whole society. Particular fields of power serve as original sites and justifications for techniques of wider-ranging inspection and control. By defining and containing what is unacceptable and by erecting norms of what is acceptable, they set guides for self-regulation, the main mode in which disciplinary power operates. Foucault provided more direct representations of the generality of this new type of power. Power configured in 'hegemonic' dominations and domination was 'a general structure of power' (1981: 94, 1982: 226). Particular or local instances of power needed a general dimension in which to be effective and vice versa (1981: 99–100). Foucault also provided a more tangible general idea of power with the sketch of 'governmentality' which we considered in the last chapter.

Whether coming from below or above, or from some fusion of the two, this new type of power appears to be so pervasive and penetrative as to exclude or subordinate other types of power. Such is the common view of Foucault on power, one which he amply supported (see e.g. Poulantzas 1978: 149–51). I will return to and refine that view later but for the moment I raise its implication for law. In terms of the story so far, disciplinary power subordinates but does not displace law:

> I do not mean to say that the law fades into the background or that the institutions of justice tend to disappear, but rather that the law operates more and more as a norm, and that the judicial institution is increasingly incorporated into a continuum of apparatuses (medical, administrative, and so on) whose functions are for the most part regulatory. A normalizing society is the historical outcome of a technology of power centered on life. We have entered a phase of juridical regression in comparison with the pre-seventeenth-century societies we are acquainted with; we should not be deceived by all the Constitutions framed throughout the world since the French Revolution, the Codes written and revised, a whole continual and clamorous legislative activity: these were

the forms that made an essentially normalizing power acceptable.

(Foucault 1981: 144)

Thus far the story would accord with and lend substance to those
tales where law in its abstract generality is displaced by the
concrete particularity of administration but where it persists in
attenuated forms along with greater 'juridification'. I will briefly
explore this subordination of law to administration and orient my
account towards showing that the connection between law and
administration is one of interdependence rather than simply one
of law's dependence.

The terms in which the rule of law has been supposedly undermined are well rehearsed. The form of legal regulation giving
discretionary power to an official to determine issues in their
infinitely varying particularity is incompatible with that stability
and predictability and with that generality of application necessary
for the rule of law. The supportive story coming from the concern
with administration has it that administrative 'procedures of
normalization come to be ever more constantly engaged in the
colonization of those of law' (Foucault 1980: 107; cf. Ewald 1990).
Such procedures 'though they may be constituted by law, operate
according to criteria which, from the point of view of law, are
indeterminate' (Rose 1979: 60). 'The discourse of discipline has
nothing in common with that of law, rule, or sovereign will'
(Foucault 1980: 106). It is 'impossible to reconcile' them (Foucault 1988: 162).

At a time seen by most theorists as its beginning and incipient
apotheosis, the rule of law was said to decline with the advance of
an administration to which it was opposed. 'Our historical
gradient', says Foucault, 'carries us further and further away from
a reign of law that had already begun to recede into the past when
the French Revolution and the accompanying age of constitutions
and codes seemed to destine it for a future that was at hand'
(Foucault 1981: 89). Law, it would seem, could not fundamentally
resist the advance of scientific administration. It had no necessary
substantive content to pit against the dictates of that science on
which administration was based. It was far from a closed system
resistant to isomorphic infiltration from administration. Further,
this science was a jealous god: it was a total view, one that claimed
to render everything in political or social life explicable, or

153

potentially explicable, in its terms, leaving room for law only as technique in its cause or as one of its branches (see Habermas 1974: 60–1; Horwitz 1977: 254, 257–9). So law, even in its own apparent expansion, seems to serve increasingly as agent, accessory and support in the advance of scientific administration. In this situation law can be seen as increasingly marginalized, confined to some largely symbolic or procedural oversight of the operation of administration (cf. Galanter 1980: 19–22; Mayhew 1971; Teubner 1983).

What is more, law's decline seems assured in a certain dependence on administration. It is because of the particularistic and pervasive powers of administration that the rule of law can be maintained in its aspects of universality and equality and seen as marking out fields for free action. The rule of law would prove too delicate for a society founded on inequality and coercive authority were not individuals pre-adapted, as it were, through administration. Administration is the necessary 'dark side' of law (Foucault 1979a: 194, 222). So, if law were substantially to counteract administration, it would undercut conditions of its own existence. Further, law's dependence would seem to be set in the unity of law and administration within the modern 'scientifico-legal complex' which would find an institutional location in, for example, the state (Foucault 1979a: 23). As a prelude to refining this insistent account and exploring the endurance of the rule of law, I will look more concretely at law's dependence to see whether the boundaries enclosing law may, on their other side, begin to indicate limits to administration.

I will begin the exploration of limits by considering the impossibility of administrative law in the setting of the judicial review of administrative action, operatively the ultimate expression of the rule of law and its dominance over administration. I will look at the situation in Britain, concentrating especially on the efflorescence of judicial assertiveness over state administration in the last thirty years. Whilst judicial assertion appears to mark a more effective control of administration by law, I aim to show that this very affirmation of legal oversight has heightened the limits of law.

For law to rule there must, minimally, be legal procedures for determining whether its requirements have been met. So long as the judiciary can effectively review excesses of administration so that administrative power is kept within legally set bounds, then, wide as those bounds may be, law in some sense continues to rule.

I will take the so-called GCHQ case as an example of both the expansion of review and the confrontation with limits (*R v. The Secretary of State for Foreign and Commonwealth Affairs* ex parte *Council of Civil Service Unions* 1985 IRLR 28). This concerned the Prime Minister's broad powers to revise the conditions of employment of civil servants. The powers were used here to take away the right to belong to a trade union enjoyed by civil servants employed at the Government Communications Headquarters, an organization which provided signals intelligence for government and which was concerned with the security of military and official communications. There was some uncertainty about whether judicial review would apply because this was an exercise of the prerogative, a form of executive power once the preserve of the monarch. The House of Lords decided that prerogative powers, or some of them, could be judicially reviewed and for this reason the case has been heralded as a major advance for judicial review by such a perceptive observer as Sedley (1988: 419). So, although the Prime Minister's broad powers over civil service contracts in their terms would cover what she did, the courts did consider whether her actions met certain notions of procedural fairness usually insisted on by the reviewing judiciary. The government, however, belatedly raised the argument that a further dimension of the prerogative powers was involved, that of national security. The government claimed that since the decision was made on grounds of national security the procedural requirements of fairness did not apply. The House of Lords accepted that national security was involved and that the requirements of fairness did not apply. What is more, the House held that it was for the government and not for courts to decide whether the interests of national security outweighed the procedural requirements.

What is significant for my purposes is the reason for this judicial abdication. To put it most simply, 'the judicial process is unsuitable for reaching decisions on national security' (GCHQ 32). Certain prerogative powers, of which only instances were given, are not 'susceptible to judicial review because their nature and subject matter is such as not to be amenable to the judicial process' (GCHQ 39). There were other statements to the same effect, one of which came from Lord Diplock (at 36). His involvement was especially significant because of the leading part he played along with Lord Reid in the expansion of the judicial review of administrative action. Lord Reid has also considered that the judiciary is excluded from reviewing certain areas 'proper' to government (see e.g. *Chandler v. Director of Public Prosecutions* 1964 AC 763 at 791). I take Lords Diplock and Reid as leading figures and GCHQ as a leading case to indicate that judicial restraint is characteristic. In all, then, the rule of law is subject to a small technical qualification. To adapt Carlyle's boast, no 'man', no matter how high he be, is above the law, so long as his excesses can be brought within the varying and uncertain bounds of what judges consider proper to their function.

Such seemingly exceptional restraint at the extremities of judicial review serves to present its normal exercise as essentially unrestricted, but it also serves to show that there is an indistinguishable normal mode of restraint. Cases of judicial review frequently contain a statement that the integrity of the administrative power being reviewed must be respected because of its exclusive expertise. There are always areas the judiciary is not fit to enter. Fashions delimiting these are varied and changeable. It is often said that review cannot be concerned with the merits or substance of an administrative decision but only with the question whether it was within the jurisdiction or powers of the official making it. It is often also said that judicial review cannot be concerned with what is decided but only with the way in which the decision is made – with, for example, whether it was made for a proper purpose or made by taking only relevant considerations into account. These are but a few of the active ingredients of the basis of judicial review, but they are sufficient to indicate what in practice has proved to be the persistent irresolution, the absence of tangible content of the judicial power in this area. This result created by the judges enables them to maintain a fluid and intangible division between law and administration, one which does not set general and enduring limits to either. Law's inevitable limits are thus dissipated and law can still be seen to rule. Judicial review is incapable of resolution or explicit consolidation. It lacks coherence and the ability to place general controls on administration (Galligan 1982). In some types of cases, judges tend toward 'sanctifying and immunising' the realm of administrators (Sedley 1987: 10), but in others they will refuse to recognize the existence of an administrative expertise (see e.g. *Bromley LBC v. GLC* 1982 2 WLR 62). Operative limits have, then, to be located outside the terms of law. A starting point could be to look at who succeeds and who fails in judicial review. It would seem that, despite the general advance of judicial review, many who are socially disadvantaged or marginalized can expect little from it (see Sedley 1987).

In short, for all the limits on law's ability to subordinate administration, it does retain a capacity to do so but one that is not testable. It is not testable in practice because the legal terms in which 'control' of administration is effected are indefinite. Such terms, characteristically, take the form of open judicial discretion. If law's ability here could be definitively tested, and its limits in relation to administration thus exposed, law could no longer lay claim to universal rule and, as the rule of law, it would cease to exist. Further, the indefinite terms of legal 'control' enable law to be responsive to the integrity and demands of administration, and it is so responsive. Law can always potentially control yet fundamentally accept the dictates of administration and not be found out for its shortcomings.

I will illustrate and expand these arguments by drawing on one remarkable line of cases within the expansion of judicial review: those dealing with disciplinary hearings in prison. The cases move from the explicit judicial recognition of law's limits to the assertion of the dominance of the rule of law. Paradoxically, the very assertion of the rule of law results, I hope to show, in law's becoming more complicit with administration. This conclusion serves as a prelude to an exploration of the symbiotic connections between law and administration.

There has been a radical reversal in the judicial review of disciplinary hearings in prisons. These hearings are conducted either by the governor of the prison or by a Board of Visitors whose members come from outside the prison. The hearings cover disciplinary charges against prisoners and complaints by them. The judicial position until recently was that such hearings were matters of domestic discipline and, at least in the case of hearings before the governor, administrative or managerial as well. As such it was not, to take a typical justification, 'the business of the courts to interfere'. The practical reasons were robustly reduced by Lord Denning in these terms: 'if the courts were to entertain actions by disgruntled prisoners, the governor's life would be made intolerable' (*Becker v. Home Office and another* 1972 2 QB 407 at 418). Beginning with *R v. Hull Prison Board of Visitors*, ex parte *St Germain* (1979 2 WLR 42), the courts have subjected these hearings to judicial review. But there remain limits which are more eloquent about what law does not cover than about what it does. This line of cases involved claims by prisoners that the requirements for procedural fairness provided for in judicial review – the requirements of 'natural justice' – should extend to these disciplinary hearings. The courts have held that natural justice does so extend in general. But they have often held that it does not so extend in particular. As with the rest of judicial review, judges have used open, obfuscating discretions and an unfettered evaluation of the nature of the administrative decisions to decide if a particular requirement of natural justice is applicable. To take the example of a case dealing with the decision of a Parole Board: it was held that natural justice did not oblige the Board to give reasons for its refusal of a prisoner's application to be released on licence because of 'the interests of society at large, including the due administration of the parole system' as Lord Denning put it (*Payne v. Lord Harris of Greenwich and another* 1981 2 All ER 842 at 846).

Although Lord Denning's incomparable bluntness may say everything needful about the inviolability of administration and its ultimate subordination of law, I will attempt to refine matters by looking at the decision of the House of Lords in *R v. Board of Visitors of HM Prison, The Maze*, ex parte *Hone* (1988 AC 379) as delivered by Lord Goff of Chieveley. The over-optimistic prisoner in this case claimed that natural justice conferred a right to be represented before the Board of Visitors. Lord Goff recognized that in a criminal court 'any person charged with a crime (or the equivalent thereof)' could claim representation (at 391). But there could be no such general right for prisoners in hearings before Boards of Visitors dealing with 'the equivalent' of a crime. A general right was not appropriate for a body, like the Board, 'exercising a disciplinary jurisdiction' (at 392). (Conferring general rights does not accord with an open judicial discretion void of content and operating on the bounds between law and administration.) In a piece of unwitting truth-telling, Lord Goff could 'see no basis' for requiring representation 'in every case as of right. Everything must depend on the circumstances of the particular case'. 'To hold otherwise', he went on to say, 'would result in wholly unnecessary delays in many cases . . . and . . . wholly unnecessary waste of time and money, contrary to the public interest' (at 392). This empathy for administration merges into deference with the climactic reason for denying representation even where the hearing involves 'the equivalent' of a crime:

Indeed, to hold otherwise . . . would . . . lead to an adventitious distinction being drawn between disciplinary offences which happen also to be crimes and those which happen not to be so, for the punishments liable to be imposed [for offences against discipline under the prison administrative rules] do not depend upon any such distinction.

(at 392)

Lord Goff bolstered these arguments by invoking the position of the prison governor. Although, in a pathbreaking statement, he made the governor's disciplinary hearings subject to natural justice, he went on to say:

The jurisdiction exercised by the Governor is of a more summary nature [than that exercised by the Board of Visitors], and should properly be exercised with great expedition . . . . In the nature of things, it is difficult to imagine that the rules of natural justice would ever require legal representation before the Governor.

(at 392)

Again there is judicial empathy and the givenness of administration, now embedded indistinguishably in the very 'nature of things'. It is this mythic nature of things that I will now investigate.

These cases illustrate a contradiction which, as we saw, inhabits judicial review in general – a contradiction between the rule of law and the imperatives of administration. Within the cases, the contradiction is resolved by the exercise of an apt discretion, in both senses of the word, entailing deference to the nature of things, to an ultimate order which judges will not disturb apart from occasional, quixotic declamations like *fiat justitia, pereat mundus* (let there be justice though the world perish). Outside of the cases, a kind of institutional fraud sustains that resolution. It limits the cases law recognizes and the cases it can recognize. The number of cases of judicial review and the resources devoted to it are infinitesimal in the scale of the number of cases of disciplinary hearings in prisons let alone the scale of state administration in general. In addition to cost, complexity, uncertainty and all the other invariant restraints on access to courts, judicial review has its own barrier erected in the process of applying for judicial review. At a preliminary stage, judicial discretion is used to filter out the bulk of cases in terms of 'criteria that are uncertain, have not been

159

openly debated or agreed and which are not widely and publicly promulgated' (Sunkin 1987: 466).

The administrative field also enforces its own practical rationalities in ways that obviate or prevent recourse to law. The governor of a prison, to continue with our example, has an obvious interest in ensuring that, in the view of one governor, disciplinary hearings have the effect of securing control, 'because in a prison, ultimately, authority has to win' (Phillips 1981: 13). Boards of Visitors pose no significant challenge to that authority. Members are appointed by the Home Secretary on the advice of prison governors and Boards. In terms of a story often told, they are dependent on authority in the prison and inevitably responsive to it (Watson 1980). Authority is further reinforced by the secrecy of the hearings. With this kind of closure around authority, as one Board member sees it, 'the rules of natural justice are not really an adequate protection against arbitrary and unfair decisions' (Watson 1980: 463).

Such authorities of delimitation, to borrow the phrase from Foucault (1972: 41–2), restrict resort to contrary authority for they contain within themselves that which is normally right and proper 'in the nature of things'. The scope remaining for law consists in a dealing with aberrations. Law is thence responsibly self-limiting. As an institution it constitutes itself and its interventions as occasional and discontinuous. Law is not, however, simply responsive to the nature of things. It evokes and affirms, even creates the normal and authority as normal. Through law's shaping and dealing with the exceptional and the aberrant, with what is outside the properly administered world, administration is rendered normal and right. Law need only correct the disturbance of things in their course and reassert the nature of things. The prescriptions of administration are mythically elevated to the realm of the given and natural by law as its proxy (cf. Barthes 1973: 129). Law, in short, provides a 'guarantee that everything really is so' (see Althusser 1971: 169). For the rule of law in liberal society, no element of personal power must come between law and the subject. The authority of administration can only be recognized as that which inexorably is, as the nature of things. Law is ultimately subordinated to an inescapable positivism which it thus serves to create. But through now exploring the nature of things yet more closely, I hope to show that this seemingly superordinate reality cannot exist itself without law.

A brief history of administration as reality:

As religion gave way to law as the principal source of social cohesion, and law to social therapy, the governing classes no longer attempted to mediate their pretensions with appeals to legitimacy. They appealed only to the unmediated authority of fact. They asked not that the citizen or worker submit to legitimate authority but that he submit to reality itself.

(Lasch 1977: 23)

Such a reality was definitively marked by the 'sciences of man and society' which emerged with administration and provided means and justifications for observing, measuring and evaluating human behaviour (Foucault 1970: chapter 10). Administrative power and knowledge are integral: they 'directly imply one another' (Foucault 1979a: 27). Taking up with Foucault again, 'in the end, we are judged, condemned, classified, determined in our undertakings, destined to a certain mode of living or dying, as a function of the true discourses which are the mirrors of the specific effects of power' (1980: 94). Power in these terms can penetrate the depths of individual being, 'into the very grain' (1980: 39), and yet extend through the whole of society. It can be intensive and extensive (see Mann 1986: 7–10).

Whether, in terms of an intense debate, power for Foucault is thus inescapable is a little beside my point. This type of power entails a claim to correspondence with reality. To know that reality is to make an inevitable power manifest. But this knowledge operating in terms of science is not complete. There are, as well, those recalcitrant enough to resist reality. These deficits are accommodated in myths of progress and in law. More of that shortly. The prime condition for the efficacy of knowledge in the cause of power is acceptance of it, not just by superordinate operatives, but by those 'judged, condemned, classified, determined' who are themselves operatives, 'always in the position of simultaneously undergoing and exercising' power (Foucault 1980: 98). In the canons of progress, belief has been replaced by knowledge. But belief has, rather, been succeeded by belief – a belief now grounded in popular empiricism and 'fact' as a 'folk-concept' (MacIntyre 1981: 76–7). This involves an acceptance of given knowledge, of factuality, rather than a participation in its production. Such participation is reserved to varieties of 'objective' or 'scientific' experts and managers. The 'individual labourer', Marx

161

says, is estranged from 'the intellectual potentialities of the labour process in the same proportion as science is incorporated in it as an independent power' (Marx 1959: 645).

The paradox of being so included in, yet excluded from, reality is resolved in mythic and magical forms of authority. The 'sciences of man and society' take original force from heroes of knowledge and discipline whose discoveries render the transcendent potential of knowledge operative in the profane world (see e.g. Zilboorg and Henry 1941). Varieties of priest–rulers give effect to such revelations. These are the agents of reality whose claimed effectiveness is 'among the central moral fictions of the age' (MacIntyre 1981: 71). Foucault captures their role in a few pages of *Madness and Civilization* where he deals with 'the apotheosis of the *medical personage*' in the history of the asylum (1967: 269 – his emphasis). The mythic heroes of discipline founding the asylum were thought to have 'opened the asylum to medical knowledge'; however, 'they did not introduce science, but a personality, whose powers borrowed from science only their disguise, or at most their justification' (1967: 271):

If the medical personage could isolate madness, it was not because he knew it, but because he mastered it; and what for positivism would be an image of objectivity was only the other side of this domination.

(Foucault 1967: 272)

This 'objectivity was from the start a reification of a magical nature, which could only be accomplished with the complicity of the patient himself' (Foucault 1967: 276). That complicity entailed 'respect and obedience' (1967: 272). Respect, we could say, is necessary because for magic to be effective the patient must respect it and cannot be 'in the know', cannot be in a position to evaluate the connection, or lack of it, between magical action and claimed outcomes. More than obedience is involved, we could say, for two reasons. For the rule of law, as we saw earlier, power had to be depersonalized. This is also the case for liberal society in general. Administration is there recognized, just as it is evoked by law, as that which inexorably is – as the nature of things. For the equality of liberalism to combine with the inequality of administration, administration is rendered in terms of positive, inevitable reality. The administered subject, then, not only obeys but is brought to believe in the credentials of the agents of reality. If we are, in Sartre's terms, condemned to be free (Sartre 1956), then we are also condemned to believe. The second and related reason why more than obedience is involved is because the compliance of the administered subject consists not just in the acceptance of repression but in the constitution of identity, 'in the very grain', in conformity with power. Modern administration, as we saw in the last chapter, provides techniques which render everyone notable in their individuality, which produce the individual as a normal, sound character (Foucault 1979a: 191–3). These techniques are characteristically oriented towards the creation of a 'voluntary' self-responsibility on the part of the subject. The individual so constituted is the indispensable conduit for the purchase of administration.

I will now connect administration as reality with law in such a way as to identify the power of law in its relation to administration. Although Foucault considered that law was 'utterly incongruous' with disciplinary power, that 'the discourse of discipline has nothing in common with that of law, rule, or sovereign will', and that 'against this ascent of a power that is tied to scientific knowledge, we find there is no solid recourse available to us today', he also indicated that 'the powers of modern society are exercised through, on the basis of, and by virtue of, this very heterogeneity between a public right of sovereignty and a polymorphous disciplinary mechanism' (1980: 106–7, 1981: 89). I shall develop that intimation of law's inevitability.

ADMINISTRATION AND THE INEVITABILITY OF LAW

Law, as we saw, evokes and confirms administration as the nature of things. That evocation is grounded in varieties of science which are at best justifications for types of magic authority wielded by such as the expert and the manager. In its operation as science, administration is limited. Law transcends these limits, mediating between the gross claims of scientific administration to match the nature of things and operative limits. In this, law does not simply enter from the outside, as it were, to compensate for the uncharacteristic and occasional shortcomings of scientific administration. Law, in its relation to administration, is itself a creative element of an ordered and ordering reality. In the result, law is not so much subordinate to administration as mythically integrated with it in a 'scientifico-legal complex' (cf. Foucault 1979a: 23). I will now expand these lines of argument.

Science, operating in the cause of administration, has to be perceived as 'objective' and apolitical (Habermas 1971: chapter 6). But science is perpetually subject to self-revelation as political or personal rule through the application of its own epistemological standards. These same standards mean that the claims of science in general to any autonomous constitution of fact must remain contingent on its 'progress' as knowledge and its self-revising discoveries. Nor does science lay claim to a full and settled knowledge of any particular, existing situation. Administration, in all, has to depend on a voluntary acceptance by its subjects beyond the claims of scientific knowledge. If scientific administration were to extend beyond the voluntary adherence of its subjects, and if it had yet to present itself and secure its own operative effects, it could not for long avoid the revelation of its political or its coercively regulating nature. Even short of these types of limiting revelation, there would remain areas where the dominance of science is not accepted and recalcitrants not prepared to submit to the rule of its operatives or to the necessity of fact. Recalcitrance can be endemic here. Take the now close to egregious case of the failure of the penitentiary. To remain an origin and site of social regulation, the penitentiary depends on its basis in crime. Not only does it fail to eliminate criminality, it goes further by creating and sustaining criminality (Foucault 1979a: 264–92). Quite apart from the creation of varieties of recalcitrance, the normal self-administering subject also has to be 'free' to take on the dictates of scientific administration. So an ability to resist these dictates, to cause science to fail, has to be recognized and dealt with. In such situations, science cannot be simply interpreted and applied. It has to be enforced.

The operative, regulatory coverage of science is limited not only by its 'internal' rationality: there are also limits to how much of the world science covers. As yet, science operates short of the full perfection of knowledge and short of the full perfection of order. There is more than a simple shortfall involved here. There are also problems of diversity. Other mythic heroes arrive on the scene creating order:

> The 'people' (the nation, or even humanity), and especially their political institutions, are not content to know – they

legislate. That is, they formulate prescriptions that have the status of norms. They therefore exercise their competence not only with respect to denotative utterances concerning what is true, but also prescriptive utterances with pretensions to justice.

(Lyotard 1984: 31)

The 'sciences of man and society' themselves do not occupy an homogenous, uniformly bounded realm. There is more a loose confederation of distinct entities and even within each there is proper scientific dispute and controversy. These sciences, in all, have no overarching mode of determination, nor can one of them move definitively to override another.

Law does not simply supplement a predominant order of administration; it presents an alternative yet complementary order. There is 'law's truth' (Nelken 1989). Order has to be rendered in such terms as 'fairness, justice, acceptability and practicality', considerations 'which may have little or no application to science' (Nelken 1989: 21), but which are central to law, not least in mediating between science and its limits in operation. Law's truth will thence often differ from the truth of science. The age of criminal responsibility, for example, may in law be expediently uniform, whereas scientific assessments of it would inevitably be varied (see Nelken 1989: 92–3).

In its relation to scientific administration, law defines and provides bounds and modes of order. The most obvious point at which law marks the frontiers of order is in bringing coercion to bear on the reluctant or recalcitrant subject who resists the dictates of science. With convenient necessity, the rule of law would say that such coercive interventions and restraints can only be legitimately effected through law. Apparatuses of legal supervision exist to enforce law's primacy in this. As we saw in the case of judicial review, the indefinite nature of the terms of legal supervision enables law to be at the same time responsive to the demands and rationalities of administration. Law can always potentially control yet fundamentally accept administration in its coercive aspect and not be 'found out' for its shortcomings. It thus incorporates administration in its coercive aspect within the rational sensibility of 'bourgeois order' and 'the sacred limits of its ethic' (cf. Foucault 1967: 58).

Whilst no longer claiming to encompass such an order, law still recognizes and, in part, constitutes its components and sets them in place. Law creates the legal subject as an effective actor, a legal subject corresponding largely to the subject of administration, as we saw in the last chapter. This subject occupies a sphere seen as private and it is only somewhat overstating the case to say that: 'as far as expectations *vis-à-vis* the administrative system are concerned, civil privatism is determined by traditions of bourgeois formal law' (Habermas 1976: 76). Administration is not excluded from this sphere but its entry is mediated through the subject. In the terms we explored in chapter 4, this 'voluntary' involvement of the subject in administration, the deep complicities between our acceptance of its dictates and the conditions of our 'freedom', mark the characteristic application of administrative power. The private sphere does not fuse indistinguishably with administration. For administration to be effective in and through it, the private sphere has to sustain a distinct vitality (see Donzelot 1980: 94). Such a distinct vitality is secured in law. According to the rule of law, it is only through law that the subject can be constrained and the sphere of the private coercively entered. The subject can take legal action, such as judicial review, to ensure that this constraining power is exercised within the bounds of law. In all, power is presented through law as a negative constraint brought into effect by transgression, thus leaving intact a realm of the subject's free action. In this way, the operation of administration is 'concealed' and rendered 'acceptable': 'the system of right is . . . designed to eliminate the fact of domination' and, we could add, designed to maintain the domination of fact (Foucault 1980: 95, 105, 1981: 86, 144).

Coercive or potentially coercive administrative power operates in a 'public' sphere which takes identity in opposition to the private. In this public sphere, law empowers scientific administration and serves to constitute it operatively. It empowers various agents of reality, various officials and practitioners, enabling them to subordinate the subject to administration. It defines, or empowers an agent of reality to define, the situations and deficiencies justifying intervention. It forms, or empowers such an agent to form, norms to be followed by the subject. The administered reality which law thus brings into existence is also affirmed in its normality through law, since judicial review of the actions of agents of reality need only be occasional and need only deal with their excesses. Law protects administration against people as well as people against administration. In all this, law gives operative content to an allowable reality not just by enacting what is within it but also by marking that which is without. Definitive bounds to the sacred order are no longer set in terms of heresy but in terms of illegality, madness and other abnormalities constituted in law. Law engages with and seeks perpetually to overcome the deviance which it creates.

Finally, law provides coherence and ultimate resolution to the varied voices of scientific administration. As transcendent sovereign, as the rule of law, law assumes a general range no less extensive in its potential effect than the operation of 'the sciences of man and society'. Modern law, having eschewed any intrinsic commitment to fact and having become inherently changeable, cannot be hindered in its responsiveness to administration by any enduringly necessary content of its own. True, the rule of law does involve a constituent commitment to depersonalized rule but, as we saw earlier, law's commitment to such rule accords with its confirmation of administration as the nature of things. As well as being in a position of responsiveness to scientific administration, law brings a cohering power to bear on it. This coherence is achieved in the mythic centralization of law-as-sovereign and its separation from 'lesser' orders over which it assumes dominance. Law thence provides a focus and a framework encompassing and demarcating the varied and discrete operations of scientific administration. This is done without bringing these operations into corrosive comparison with each other. Such a comparison would reveal their uncertain and overlapping bounds and challenge their claims to autonomy. Since law is a distinct and different order which relates fields of scientific administration to each other, these fields are protected from a disintegrating competition within the dimension of science. The legal demarcation and separation of these fields is enforced through judicial review – through such requirements as that administrative power has to be exercised for its 'proper purpose' or be exercised only in the light of 'relevant' considerations. The massive sum of scientific administration and its extensively shaping effect on the subject is masked in this dispersal of it through law. Requirements within judicial review for reasonableness and fairness in the exercise of administrative power serve to unify and present administration in terms of restraint and neutrality. The small price paid by administration for all this is a marginal abdication in favour of 'law's truth' of its extensive hold on reality.

I will now draw all this together in terms of a mythic mutuality. The Benthamite dream of reconciling law and administration in perfect order is an impossible one because, says Foucault, the effort to fulfil it leads to the integration of law into administration (Foucault 1988: 162). Others would mark or foretell the death or retreat of law in the advance of administration. My initial focus on law through administration confirmed and reinforced the story of demise or decline in part. Law, as the rule of law, was seen to depend integrally on administration. Even in its claims to supervise and control administration, law was responsive and labile in its accommodation of administration. And even its claim to an enduring distinction in terms of fair and objective process served to constitute an impermeable administration as 'the order of things'.

The story of the death of law is, however, one told in small circles. The conundrum posed at the outset involved the survival of law in the face of the persistence, even the expansion, of administration. Administration, as we saw, depended on law to mediate between its constituent universal claims and its operative limits. This law accorded with the claims of the rule of law to combine an encompassing or universal rule with sustaining areas of the subject's free action. It would be inaccurate, not to say unwise, to extract from this a perduring capacity of law to stand securely in favour of the individual or the market in the face of administration. As far as my analysis went in its confinement to the mythic relation between the two, law and administration are mutually supportive, even, or especially, when they are in opposition. Law, as operatively limited, evokes and relies on a scientific administration in all its mythic purity, as the very nature of things, set beyond the doubts and diversities that compromise it in operation. In its operative dimension, administration evokes and relies on a law no less rarefied in its mythic purity. This law is, in the jurisprudential sense, a normative order distinct from administration and dominant over it. For its part, administration thus confirms the autonomy of law and the transcendent universality of its rule. This was not a law restrained by its relation to administration, much less a law which administration infiltrates and comprehensively undermines. But there is point to stories of law's decline in the advance of administration. The nature of things does not provide a firm boundary where law's rule can decently stop in the face of the inevitability of the nature of things. This nature is infinitely varied and changing. It is operatively constituted in varieties of thaumaturgic decree by the agents of reality. In accepting these as the nature of things, law subordinates itself to administration. Yet law retains its mythic purity by investing its own subaltern thaumaturge, the judge, with power over the terms of that acceptance, a power in the form of necessarily indefinite discretion. In the maintenance of purity, borders become perilous places (Douglas 1970). The integrity and identity of law are here at risk. They are preserved ultimately in the mutual and mythic complicity between law and administration. Each takes on what is displaced but remains operatively integral in the constitution of the other.

POPULAR JUSTICE

A reciprocal compensation is also to be found in my second example of the mutuality of myths, one linking law with what is most compendiously called popular justice. Proponents of popular justice see it as 'alternative' to law and as constituted in opposition to law. Its detractors see it as a sympathetic extension of law, as indistinguishable from it. In terms of its myth of origin, popular justice is set against a formal and an alienated realm from which it is essentially different and apart. With its constriction and artifice, this realm is contrasted with the more spontaneous, nature-like, intrinsically human characteristics of popular justice. Such a realm is occupied by formal law and administration. But closer observation of popular justice reveals compatibilities, even similarities, between it and these formal modes of regulation. This could be explained, as in so many accounts, by reducing popular justice to these formal modes. Popular justice is but an extension of formal regulation, its mere mask or agent. In terms of my argument, there is point to seeing popular justice and law as both opposed and integral. The conflict is accommodated by the mythic mutuality between law and popular justice which I now explore (see also Fitzpatrick 1992).

The supposed retreat from formal regulation to a private realm or community is nowadays so extensive and so often manifestly spurious as to make a general scepticism obligatory. The first batch of alternatives, offered mainly in the 1970s, were mediation and other types of dispute settlement alternative to traditional courts as well as 'community' adaptations of penal and psychiatric regulation. These exercises provoked fierce academic debate. On one side, the informal and sites of the informal were attributed a distinct, even autonomous identity. On the other side, the informal and its sites were denied such an identity and reduced essentially in terms of some other surpassing identity such as legal regulation by the state (see Fitzpatrick 1988b: 179–82). This resort to supposed alternatives broadened in the 1980s with neo-liberal adoptions of 'private' modes replacing or reducing state regulation, a shift accompanied by the expansion of that regulation in its functions of explicit control of the individual. All this has heightened the perception of revived communities and other particular groupings, natural and spontaneous in their self-regulation which is akin to custom and opposed to law.

Popular justice takes identity through the mythic mode in which negative opposition provokes and produces positive contents. The great figure of opposition and rejection is the state. 'Alternative' justice is set in a dynamic of opposition to the formalized and centralized power of the state. This justice exists in the denial or partial dissolution of state power, or it exists in the operative affirmation of the limits of such power. Even where alternative justice works specifically in conjunction with state power, it does so on the basis that such power is limited and that alternative justice makes good this deficiency. Alternative justice does what the state cannot. As a type of state power, formal law has proved the most productive affront to popular justice (cf. Nader 1988). Formal law focuses on delimited and pre-defined types of behaviour separated from any extensive context. Existential involvement of the subject is absent or restricted to straitened conceptions of responsibility. Popular justice takes identity in positive contrast to all this. It is concerned with the whole person and no case is specifically confined at the outset in its social relations. Being so unconfined, popular justice can make its characteristic claims to reflect, or strengthen, or even create an holistic 'community'.

Establishing the particular mythic mutuality between popular justice and law, showing that each takes on what is integral to but denied in the other, involves locating elements of formal law in a site that foundationally rejects it. Teasing them out requires searching in the operative details of popular justice. In doing this, we would have to avoid those common situations where popular justice is formally joined to legal modes since the operative details could be infected by law. To meet the combination of purity and available detail, I will resort to the setting of the United States and the Community Boards of San Francisco, relying considerably on DuBow's unpublished evaluation of them (1987a). The mere singularity of an instance forced by the demand for detail is somewhat made up for by the Board's having had a large influence in the growth of popular justice and, in particular, having provided a model for numerous other programmes (Harrington and Merry 1988: 918). I will also provide more extensive evidence for key points.

A considerable literature on Community Boards, or providing their foundational ideas, abundantly attests to their being conceived as profoundly 'alternative' to the state, especially to state law (DuBow 1987c: 35). The Boards stand opposed to the alienating professionalism of the state, to its formality and its 'record-keeping apparatus', to its insensitivity in the face of the real needs of individuals and communities, and to its illimitable arrogation of conflicts and other matters that can only be dealt with adequately by individuals and neighbourhoods (Shonholtz 1984: 5–7, 15, 21–2). Resort to the state 'suppresses and evades' conflict 'in its full interactive dynamic', drastically narrows the range of matters considered relevant to it and renders these matters manipulable; in doing all this, the state undermines the responsibility of the individual and the neighbourhood for conflict and destroys 'the vitality of individual and community life' (Shonholtz 1984: 2, 4, 8, 13). So individual and communal self-reliance oppose the intrinsic assumptions of state regulation (Shonholtz 1984: 17, 21).

These originating assertions are reflected in the practice and strategies of the Community Boards. The responsibility of individuals for their conflict and its resolution is to be inculcated and in this way the authenticity of the disputing process will be secured. Thus, the Boards claim a significance which sets them apart from other forms of alternative justice in their refusal to accept cases where an agency of the legal system retains jurisdiction: the continuing pressure of the legal system can produce a 'less authentic' result (DuBow 1987c: 5). Comparable pressure from the Panels which hear disputes must, of course, also be avoided. The 'defined passivity' of the Panels, their eschewing 'active intervention', leaves space for the authenticity of the parties to operate (DuBow 1987c: 50). There is a 'practice of minimal intervention based on the principle that the disputants are responsible for resolving their own dispute' (DuBow 1987c: 53). Again, 'the conflict belongs to the disputants; any resolution is of their own making' (DuBow

171

1987c: 50). Disputants are considered holistically and only the authentic resolution of their conflict promoted, even if this may mean having authenticity thrust upon them. The prime emphasis of the Panels is to extract the feelings of the parties, so much so that there is a 'functional tendency to concentrate on the feelings of the parties rather than on the facts in the dispute' (DuBow 1987c: 56). Thus, in one case, there was a 'pronounced attempt by the Panel to concentrate on the feelings of the parties when both of them were more concerned about the issues of money and responsibility' (DuBow 1987c: 58). So the handbook for training conciliators to serve on Panels contrasts their role with that of mediators in other programmes in this way:

> if racism or sexism became apparent on the part of the disputants, a mediator might de-emphasize these issues to avoid inflaming hostility and to reach an agreement more efficiently. The conciliator [sic], on the other hand, would identify these attitudes and encourage their expression, to promote greater understanding, since these factors can significantly affect the quality of a relationship.
>
> (Hawkins 1986: 6)

The responsibility and the vitality of the neighbourhood are less precisely articulated in strategies and in practice than those of the individual. 'Neighborhood building' is a 'central goal' of Community Boards, as is 'developing a neighborhood's capacity to respond to neighborhood disputes' (DuBow 1987b: 1). There would seem to be nothing assuredly linking the Boards' core activity of dispute handling with these desiderata.

Bare and preliminary as it is, my account of popular justice begins to show that it is not constituted only in opposition to the formal. Panels seem to exercise a formal power that is inextricable to and yet more basic than the informal or the popular, more fundamental than the authentic participation of the parties. In mapping the operation of power within popular justice, an exemplary beginning is provided by Harrington and Merry in their telling general observations of alternative justice (1988: 726–9). As I interpret these observations, mediators see their own purposive strategies as the prime impetus and basis for their activity (see also Dingwall 1988). So, although responsiveness to the parties is emphasized, it is a responsiveness contained within such strategies, within modes of manipulation and direction that operate beyond the knowledge of the parties. Thus, parties can be induced to engage with each other through the manoeuvring of eye contact. Or the confidence of the parties is to be purposively created. They are to be made to feel that they are being listened to and that their concerns count. In a 'successful' case, parties are brought to accept, to take on themselves, a reality of which the mediator is agent. Yet the parties are seen as ultimately responsible. The door through which they can depart the scene remains open. But this standard picture ignores what is waiting outside the door – a reality of coercive aspects which is invoked by the mediators in order to promote 'agreement'. I do not mean this egregious interpretation to say any more than it does. It does not, for example, impute ulterior motives to mediators. What it says about the orientation and dynamics of informal dispute resolution is just the way things are and I am extracting from it 'the nature of things'.

In DuBow's predominantly sympathetic evaluation, a Panel derives power from identifying with the process used in hearings:

> However neutral it may be with respect to the dispute that it hears, it is an advocate of CB and its process. When it is most faithful to its advocacy of that process, thereby avoiding the kind of control that professional mediators, lawyers, or courts might exercise, the Panel unwittingly employs coercion through its unyielding implementation of the process.
>
> (DuBow 1987c: 69)

And he asks:

> What is the essential makeup of the CB Panel? What is the core of its identity? First, it is a group of neighbors who carry the four-phase CB hearing process, and it is very self-conscious about upholding that process, sometimes to the point of being legalistic.
>
> (DuBow 1987c: 49)

In the first two of these four, set phases, the parties express their perceptions of the issues and their feelings. They are thus 'encouraged' to communicate with each other. In the third phase – 'sharing responsibility for the conflict and its resolution' – 'the parties are now guided through an understanding of their responsibility in both the existence of the conflict and the resolution'. Finally, the resolution 'is clearly spelled out', 'an agreement form' is concluded, and 'the hearing is closed' (Shonholtz 1984: 18).

173

Informal and responsive as parts of the process may appear to be, it does have, in all, powerful, defining and organizing effects. Thus, in one case:

> The Panel was so taken with its responsibility to the CB process that it tended to ignore the attitudes of the parties, and it tended to miss opportunities to use information from the hearing to advance toward resolution of the conflict.
>
> (DuBow 1987c: 58)

And in another case:

> As a proxy for the CB process, the panel seemed at first to be trying to prevent a resolution from coming too soon, since there are three Phases prior to the resolution. In that sense it tended to break off communication between the parties when they wanted to discuss the technical details of a plan they could agree to. It also tried to get the Parties to communicate about underlying feelings and issues when there evidently were none.
>
> (DuBow 1987c: 61)

An 'intervention technique' used in training Panel members in a mock hearing directs the trainer 'to make sure that people are clear that what they are trying to do coincides with the purpose of the phase, ask team members what phase they are in and what are its objectives' (Hawkins 1986: 55). An effective technique, apparently, for 'the common occurrence of panelists trying to identify which Phase the hearing is in is a major instance of the form of a process displacing the demands of a dispute itself' (DuBow 1987c: 71). The four-phase process, as I will now show, is only one of a number of inevitable organizing elements which constitute this mode of popular justice as a formed site of power.

No matter what its unique virtues, the Community Board hearing does share with other types of alternative justice organizing elements contributing to an operative core of formal power. Its quasi-litigious focus and its 'defined passivity' accord a formal equality of power to the parties that can deny significant inequalities between them (see e.g. DuBow 1987c: 53, 58). That same focus means that a Panel has 'no mechanism for engaging the program in a larger social issue unearthed by a two-party dispute' (DuBow 1987c: 50). There is even an understandable tendency to avoid such connections and legalistically to confine the dispute to the issues and forms in hand (see e.g. DuBow 1987c: 54). These forms and modes are reinforced as a professional orientation on the part of members of Panels and by their general cohesion. They often see their training and their work in professional terms and as beneficial to their careers (DuBow 1987c: 16, 35). Training, the encouragement of 'teamwork', involvement together in the hearing process, identifying favourably with the neighbourhood, all these build up a sense of a distinct 'internal' or 'exclusive' community (DuBow 1987c: 69, 1987d: 13, 32, 41; Hawkins 1986: 39).

The foundational role of members of Panels is heightened in their being 'agents of reality'. The neutrality of Panels in the disputing process positions them to respond to a general reality beyond yet brought to bear on that process. Thus, an old woman who complains about noise can be put in perspective as either '"crazy" or . . . overreacting' (DuBow 1987c: 62). Further, 'the Panel, with its three to five persons, is literally and symbolically a public entity' (DuBow 1987c: 52). The Panel dominates the table – that most potent figure which posits a shared reality on the basis of which a dispute is resolvable. The neighbourhood provides a like figure linking the parties and the Panel. The Panel takes on a 'representative role as neighbors of the parties' embodying 'community norms and values' (DuBow 1987c: 69). In all, the 'community board model advances a community-based normative justice system. The model is premised on a community perspective' and 'the neighborhood should exercise responsibility for a conflict' (Shonholtz 1984: 13–14).

In mythic terms, the community and the individual are the fount of the informal and of the popular in alternative justice. The individual's voluntary participation and willingness to adapt and enter into agreements are the foundation of the whole process. Everything else in the process – the efficacy and role of the mediators or conciliators, its very success – depends on and springs from that involvement. Formal elements in the process can only be secondary to the thrust of this informal, popular element. My analysis would reverse this mythic picture. In that revelatory picture of mediators presented by Harrington and Merry (1988), we can discern a disputing individual who is to be manoeuvred into certain defining modes of engagement with the other party and with the mediator, an individual who is responsible yet responsive to a pre-set reality. The individual that emerges from the story-so-far of the Community Boards is not of a completely different kind. Indeed, even greater depths of individuality, extending to the very feelings of the parties, are to be appropriated and shaped in terms of the power being exercised. It is a 'basic value' of the Boards' processes 'that it is of prime importance to probe for the underlying feelings that disputants have about each other' (DuBow 1987c: 50). Feelings are elevated over facts and aspirations, even over a resolution of the dispute. The primacy of feelings disconnects the disputants from the social forces encapsulated in their conflict. At best, what is relevant is how they feel about such things. The primacy of feelings inculcates an acceptant attitude in the parties, one in which they are to be fully responsible for 'their' conflict. All of which must be heightened in the reciprocity entailed in the baring of feelings. If I bare my feelings and become vulnerable to you, almost in return you should become vulnerable to me. The vulnerability of the parties and their induced readiness to take on responsibility leaves the ground clear for the most effective powers that can occupy it, mediators and conciliators as representatives of the juridical element. In its voluntarism and assumption of limitless responsibility, the figure of the individual takes on itself and accepts as its own the effects of popular justice – effects the origins of which lie in constricted, pre-formed processes and relations of power.

It is likewise with community and neighbourhood. These provide an infinite source of standards and legitimations invoked and given effect by and within the operation of popular justice. Community and neighbourhood lay claim to an infinite disciplinary domain where power can respond to such vast and expansive imperatives as the 'potential' for 'disorder', the need for 'control', dealing with 'pre-criminal' and 'problematic' activities, and responding to community 'ideas' and 'fears' (Shonholtz 1987: 42–5). Indeed, in Shonholtz's definitive account, such categories can encompass community and neighbourhood. Thus, 'community' is equated with 'social control' and as 'the area of prevention [of conflict] is extended . . . thereby the scope of community is extended as well' (Shonholtz 1987: 47, 52).

The maintenance of the formal and law-like processes and relations of popular justice depends on the infinite, the unbounded capacities and natures of the individual and the community. I will now consider these mythic figures within popular justice more generally. They exist in a mythically elevated, depoliticized realm of original innocence. As free-floating entities, not compromised by inexorable ties to the specific, they can supportively accommodate the widest range of effects produced by popular justice. And they can do this in a way that does not challenge the formal sources of these effects or call such sources to account. The formal elements of popular justice are presented as operating within and in the cause of these whole, unalienated entities. The acceptant, responsible individual and the protean community absorb formal and juridical elements of popular justice that would otherwise be incompatible with its defining, informal attributes.

I have already considered in the last chapter the figure of the self-realizing, responsible individual taking identity through the internalizing of different modes of control. We can now add to these modes the practices of alternative justice already instanced by Community Boards and in mediation as observed by Harrington and Merry (1988: 726–9). These are indistinguishable in their instrumental, manipulative modes and inculcation of unbounded responsibility from such foundational modern systems of control as those described by Tuke in 1813 in his account of the first psychiatric asylum in England (Tuke 1964: esp. 131–86). What is particularly significant for popular justice is the equation of this self-responsible, self-ordering individual with the individual 'as posited by nature' (Marx 1973: 346). This mythic nature exists apart from the artifices of form and culture. It is spontaneous, an unbounded, authentic realm of adamic and unsullied wholeness where we can be 'truly', naturally ourselves. Its civil equivalent is the private sphere which is marked out by law but not regulated by it (O'Donovan 1985: 2–3). This is where the new individual can be left to assume responsibility for her or his own actions (O'Donovan 1985: 9). So, in theorizing about law and 'private justice', Henry relies on an 'informal, spontaneous level' (Henry 1983: 61). Or an article can be about 'alternative dispute resolution and divorce: natural experimentation in family law' (Teitelbaum and DuPaix 1988). And the natural, the authentic individual has long been situated integrally in the natural, the authentic community (Turner 1987). 'The new community justice system recruits from the neighborhoods the natural dispute resolvers' (Shonholtz 1987: 47). It is in the vacuity of the natural and the authentic that we find 'what a dispute is all about' and 'actual substantive relationships in ongoing communities' (Lempert and Sanders 1986: 478).

Tenuous traces of community supporting this mythic foundation of alternative justice have failed to survive critical explorations
of their 'substance'. But such deficiencies are hardly to the point.
The dynamic of identity does not come from mundane empirical
correspondences. It is a myth-making dynamic of rejection, of
negativity. It can be readily encapsulated in the figure of Utopia,
of no-place. The true community of informalism is a vacuous
Utopia constituted in abrupt opposition to the perceived in-
authenticity of certain existent sites of power (cf. Delgado 1987:
312–13). Like the figure of the spontaneous, unregulated individual, Utopian alternatives to the administered world prove to be
modes of further implicating us in it (Minson 1985: 111–12).
Through its identity in negation, the free-floating figure of community is able to range temporally and geographically in search of
substance, absorbing, as we have seen, imperatives of control,
discipline and pre-emptive surveillance. In one version, community is meant to provide a 'modern analogue to the historical
experience of community' in the European colonization of North
America (Shonholtz 1987: 46). But the colonized, at least elsewhere, are not left out of the picture. A voracious ethnography
provided accounts of 'different cultures' in which 'the apparent
naturalness . . . of informal dispute processing' provided ideate
origins for alternative justice in the United States (Matthews 1988:
2–3; cf. Merry 1982). The savage and the savage community, 'the
state of nature', provided pre-civilized and pre-legal origins. Such
a community in its primal innocence was a simple, consensual and
unified whole. Community was also validated in the evolutionary
history and the sociology of law which provided inverse terms for
the story of popular justice. A simple, integral community and its
justice, still retrievable in their palatable aspects, are displaced in
the complexity and differentiation of industrialized, urbanized,
legal society (see Merry 1990: 173). Confirming similarities were
found with the 'primitive' communities studied by anthro-
pologists. And these similarities correspond to those attributed to
the pre-modern community in general. But this idea of community
is a construct of the colonial experience and of the degradation of
community in transitions to capitalism. The end-result is a reduced
and contained 'native' or 'peasant' community, the diversity and
complexity of which have been denied. And it was this type of
community which provided origins for alternative justice.

This adoption of a solidary wholeness provides a foundation for the juridical in popular justice. Foucault could tie the destruction of revolutionary popular justice to its attempting to operate through the figure of the table (Foucault 1980: chapter 1). The table is an effective symbol importing the myth of law into processes of popular justice. It serves to subordinate competing claims to shared standards of general applicability. With alternative justice, the community provides a supposedly shared, consensual domain and the table continues to bring it to bear on competing claims. The terms and processes of this competition replicate the individual, professional and depoliticized bases of formal legal regulation, as the Community Boards instanced (see also Cain 1988). The figure of community thence subordinates popular justice to formal law. Community establishes a proportion with and a subordination to a wider reality. It is 'small-scale', 'decentralized' and qualitatively different to the alienated, formal world beyond it. It does not, therefore, challenge or disrupt the wider world in the terms of that world. Modern law, as an operative embodiment of the wider world, is thus readily affirmed in its constitutional opposition to and domination of lesser orders.

Law, however, depends on popular justice for its own integrity. This is partly because 'in political situations where jobs still have to be done, formalisation can never be used completely' (Bloch 1974: 65). More specifically, in its transcendent, mythic being, the rule of law asserts a competence to do, potentially, anything. Yet as myth, law is operative and thence constrained in its relation to other myths or the mundane. If the integrity of law is to be maintained, these limits on its universal competence must be kept apart from it. This is done in several significant ways and one involves the denial of explicit form to such limits. Limiting form is denied or dissipated in the ideas of the informal and the popular. Vivid examples are already available and a case study is not needed here. Thus Cain's enthralling study of court processes finds them necessarily dependent on informal modes operating 'outside' them (Cain 1986). Henry's studies of law and labour discipline provide another example (Henry 1982). The divide between law's universal pretensions and its limited purchase on the labour relation was obscured and mediated by relying on a 'private justice' in the workplace and suppressing the challenge this private justice would otherwise pose to the dominance of law and capital.

Law is associated supportively with the limits on which its formed integrity depends. Negatively, it constitutes those limits by standing in continual opposition to what they contain and affirming its essential alterity. In the Utopian response to this rejection, the popular and the informal are constituted in opposition to law. Positively, law creates such limits both by marking out a 'free', 'private' realm and by providing forms of the informal such as alternative dispute-settling modes attached to legal processes.

As with administration, I would summarize this in terms of a mythic mutuality. Popular justice takes identity in opposition to formal law, yet it is based on a core of formal, juridical power. This contradiction is mediated by the mythic figures of the individual and the community. These figures combine the attributes of formality and professed informality, founding the formal yet absorbing it into what seems an encompassing informality. The rule of law, 'the abstract formalism of legal certainty', in its turn takes identity in opposition to 'every form of "popular justice"' (Weber 1954: 351, 356). Yet the integrity of law depends on the popular justice it opposes and the informal element of law is necessarily placed apart from it. I will now conclude this chapter by elaborating on this mutuality.

THE LIMITS OF LAW

This dynamic of identity in opposition is located, I argue, in the particular position of myth in modernity. As mythic, Occidental law claims to be transcendent. This claim is made operative in law's power of centralization and sovereignty, in its opposing and dominating 'the nature of things'. Yet with modernity, reality is unitary and mundane and this particular construction of law must confront limits incompatible with its illimitable transcendence, and must subordinate its identity as different in 'the ever-to-be-accomplished unveiling of the Same' (Foucault 1970: 340). Here, I suggest, is one way of encompassing the profound and persistent jurisprudential divide explored in chapter 1 between law as autonomous and law as dependent on society. The creation of autonomous law, which we explored in chapter 3, was mythically sustained and made compatible with historicist and social claims on law in a particular myth of progression recounted in chapter 4. In that story, law as dependent on society becomes progressively autonomous in an evolutive, quasi-biological process of division and specialization. That mythology becomes somewhat 'whitened' but it persists in its dynamic terms within current social thought.

This leaves a problem of how this mythic independence and transcendence of law are to be made compatible with the limits imposed by a mundane reality or by other things aspiring to a competing mythic transcendence. In this chapter, I have shown how operative figures of a 'society' fragmented in its own evolutive mythology relate to law in ways that limit it yet sustain its transcendent being. These ways were subdued or 'whitened' versions of that template mythology in which law's differentiation and autonomy are secured in its very dependence on social forces. In the pairing of law with administration or of law with popular justice, each provided conditions for the other's integral existence, yet, in part because of this, they stood in a certain mutual autonomy and inviolability. It was not simply a matter of society entering into and forming law, as standard accounts of the relation between law and society have it, but also a matter of law entering into and forming society. But law's formative operations and functions in these sites of society are subordinated or held apart in the cause of their integrity. The presences of these other sites in law are similarly subordinated or held apart. What is more, law erects boundaries and forms of these other sites that are compatible with its own gross claims.

In creating these boundaries and forms, law itself becomes formed in ways that secure its integrity. Law's relation with administration was effected in legal terms that were indefinite – in open discretions and loose standards, such as standards of fairness and reasonableness. The resulting discretionary form of law supposedly undermines the classic rule of law, but, as we saw, it serves to protect the rule of law by avoiding its confrontation with what would undermine it. In its mutual mediation with sites of society, law constitutes them as realms of the factual, the natural or the popular, and thereby forms itself as their negation. These attributes are not simply there awaiting a facile discovery. They have to be constructed often in the face of contrary characters that can themselves be law-like.

Such a construction against the grain and such an exercise of modulated discretions call for a protective enclosed priesthood to serve and secure the myth of law. Judges are usually accorded the position of high priests as 'the living oracles' of law (Blackstone 1825: 68 – I). The whole community professionally organized around law is redolent of religion, not just in the perception of outside observers but also in its own self-presentation (Goodrich 1990: chapter 8; Sugarman 1991: 58). This priesthood arrogates to itself social tasks usually of a stunning simplicity, erecting an arcane knowledge around their supposed complexity (Konecni and Ebbesen 1984). It claims in this to speak for the people, to represent common sense and common values. What results, is an:

> Exclusion of dialogue in favour of an authoritarian mono-logue of initiation . . . a culture confined within the parameters of a professionalised and esoteric language, in turn supported by a jurisprudence of legal univocality within which the institutional meaning of the law is always already given and merely remains to be said.
>
> (Goodrich 1987: 97)

This situation is reflected and secured in the rituals which give effect to law's mythic force and identity. Ritual and the formalized language of ritual ensure the 'set apart' and insular character of an activity, the 'disconnection' and even antagonism between it 'and the real world' (Bloch 1974: 56, 77). The ritual is pre-set and 'invariant', and participants come to it from the 'outside' (Bloch 1974: 68). Although rituals are usually long-enduring, they are not impervious to the influence of participants (see e.g. Bloch 1986). So law as ritual is not simply a matter of ideal standards imposed on a populace. Nor can it be equated simply with behaviour. Rather, these dimensions, to which law is usually and variously reduced, are fused by ritual into something else which is myth. Through legal ritual, people act in accordance with certain forms to create and sustain situations that have their distinct, legal identity. As Winn so vividly illustrates, acting in conformity with legal requirements for the formation and operation of a corpora-tion or for making an arrest evokes and affirms a realm that is *sui generis* (Winn 1991). I shall in the next and final chapter consider the most influential jurisprudential settlement of that solitary realm and explore its mythic character.

6

‘

LAW AS MYTH

> The sole visible and indubitable law that is imposed upon us
> is the nobility, and must we ourselves deprive ourselves of
> that one law?
>
> (Kafka 1988a: 438)

LIFE AND LEGAL AUTONOMY

Everything up to this final chapter could be read as an elaboration
of the extravagant things I am now going to say about the supreme
text of jurisprudence, Hart's *The Concept of Law* (1961). As a
prelude to locating the exotically impure in a work that is a
by-word in the trade for purity, I will adapt a previous analysis
which identifies a profound dislocation or contradiction in the
work (Fitzpatrick 1991). I will then show how myth, in mediating
this contradiction, is essential to this most influential assertion of
law's autonomy. In the process, I will amplify those mythic evocations of law's autonomy encountered in the first chapter.

'In the English-speaking world', *The Concept of Law* now provides
'the standard position' in jurisprudence (Leith 1988: 85). From
within jurisprudence and from without, superlatives have been
showered upon it (see Moles 1987: 5). *The Concept* underlies 'Hart's
position of pre-eminence among British jurists of the twentieth
century' and his position as 'the focal figure . . . for English-
speaking jurists' (MacCormick 1981: 12, 19). It 'remains the most
significant post-war text in jurisprudence' (Lloyd and Freeman
1985: 403). It also 'remains a central focus of jurisprudence teaching in the UK', with surveys of jurisprudence teaching placing it
very much on top of the list of works used (Barnett and Yach 1985:
158–61). It retains a mythic impermeability despite, or perhaps

183

because of, the hundreds of papers that would seek to revise or undermine it. Those writers sympathetic to it have tended not to engage, or not to engage fully, with destructive criticism. The effect of their own contributions is difficult to pin down because it is usually not clear whether these contributions are revisions or exegesis (see Hart 1982: chapter X; MacCormick 1987: 105). The upshot is that both detractors and supporters still address *The Concept of Law* with its key teachings largely unchanged since its publication in 1961 (e.g. Hart 1987; Moles 1987).

There is good reason for this continuity and for the high regard in which *The Concept of Law* is held. In this book Hart restored and set new sustaining terms for a positivist jurisprudence that appeared increasingly impoverished in the face of jurisprudential tendencies which it was unable either to challenge or to contain. To sustain positivist jurisprudence, to endow it with the ability to deal with these tendencies, Hart provided it with a new foundation derived from linguistic philosophy, especially Wittgenstein in *Philosophical Investigations* (1968). This may seem a distortion because Wittgenstein's explicit part in *The Concept* is confined in two footnotes (Hart 1961: 234, 249 – page references without more will refer to this work). Hart later provided a more general acknowledgement (Hart 1983: 2–3) and I will show that Wittgenstein's influence was central.

The Concept of Law is usually seen as an exercise in linguistic philosophy, one which secured Hart's renown as a linguistic philosopher as well as a jurist (MacCormick 1981: 12–19). The first four chapters of the book are largely in the idiom of linguistic philosophy and impelled by its characteristic concern. In looking initially at Hart as linguistic philosopher, I will give references to Wittgenstein that parallel Hart's resort to that philosophy. Hart begins securely within the tradition by addressing the question of definition (see also Hart 1954b). He confronts and disposes of the old primal question, 'What is law?'. This venerable puzzle has resisted resolution because it is founded in linguistic confusion (Wittgenstein 1968: paras. 109, 119, 123). The origin of error lies in the experience of meaning which the question evokes. That is, a word like 'law' must name something to which it corresponds (Wittgenstein 1968: paras. 26–7). A word has essential or inherent meaning. One way of testing such meaning would be to match the word against some empirically observable reality. Linguistic philosophy was created in opposition to such a view of meaning and such a way of testing it. Whether words stand adequately for things was only one kind of question that could be asked about them. If we placed words in their ordinary context, if we looked at their characteristic use, we would see that they did much more than just stand for things (Wittgenstein 1968: paras. 19, 23, 146–8). So some legal realists may see law in terms of a prediction of what judges will do. But this view of law does not capture the ways in which a judge uses a legal rule 'as his *reason* and *justification* for punishing the offender' (10 – Hart's emphasis). The multiple and complex uses of 'law' cannot be reduced to a simple statement of factual correspondence – reduced, in this case, to what judges are seen to be doing. Such a statement would reflect something of what is going on but far from all of what is going on. This attempt to capture an essence of law which would be the same in all situations where the word 'law' was used has merely reduced varied and multiple uses to one possible use. Hart quotes Wittgenstein's instruction for considering various 'games' and the question of what is common to all of them (234):

> Don't say: 'There *must* be something common, or they would not be called "games"' – but *look and see* whether there is anything common to all. For if you look at them you will not see something that is common to *all*, but similarities, relationships, and a whole series of them at that.
>
> (as in Wittgenstein 1968: para. 66)

Linguistic philosophy effects its revolution by showing that perennial questions posed in philosophy disappear or can be radically recast in a more tractable form. Just so, Hart finds prior jurisprudence to be wrongly oriented. The result is a 'record of failure and there is plainly need for a fresh start' which he provides (78). The record of failure is revised by looking at characteristic contexts in which 'law' and significant legal usages appear and by considering the diversity of jobs which they do. Words and the functions they perform are seen in their particularity, described as they are and not reduced in other terms (Wittgenstein 1968: paras. 19, 23). For use and context linguistic philosophers look to language. But in the observation and evaluation of linguistic use, they also look to non-linguistic presuppositions of that use. For a judge to use a legal rule as a rule presupposed, as we saw earlier, a certain commitment to that rule. But there are limits to what can be presupposed. For linguistic philosophy use is prime and presupposition has to be necessarily related or relatable to use.

Hart brings the force of linguistic philosophy most immediately to bear on the work of John Austin, the ancestor figure of English jurisprudence. In Hart's estimation, 'Austin's influence on the development in England of the subject has been greater than that of any other writer' (Hart 1954a: xiv). Much of *The Concept* is taken up with setting Hart's own standpoint in a critique of Austin. Indeed, Austin is Hart's proper obsession. His positivist jurisprudence dominated the subject for close to a century until its displacement by *The Concept* and it still retains a position of prominence close to Hart's in jurisprudence (Barnett and Yach 1985: 159). But Hart's version of Austin is truncated, corresponding to the impoverished rendition of Austin received in jurisprudence. Austin attempted, Hart says, 'to analyse the concept of law in terms of the apparently simple elements of commands and habits' (18). And 'we shall state and criticize a position which is, in substance, the same as Austin's doctrine but probably diverges from it at certain points' (18). It certainly does diverge but that for Hart is of no significance since 'our principal concern is not with Austin but with the credentials of a certain type of theory which has perennial attractions whatever its defects may be' (18). These attractions lie in the siren call for definition, for encapsulating what law is in some factual formula such as one involving 'the apparently simple elements of command and habits' which Austin supposedly uses. But the problem is that the 'elements he uses do not include the notion of a *rule* or the rule dependent notion of what *ought* to be done' (Hart 1954a: xi–xii – his emphasis; cf. Austin 1861–3: 158–9 – I). When we see rules operating in legal contexts it becomes evident that they cannot be reduced to a correspondence with certain observable facts about commands and habits, any more than they could be reduced, as we saw earlier, to a prediction of what judges will do. What these reductions capture, at most, is how the operation of a rule could appear to an external observer. They do not capture the internal perspective of the operation of rules, the perspective of those who use and live rules. It is this perspective which is distinctive of rules and of law. Such is the next stage of Hart's argument, very much in brief, which I will now amplify and analyse.

To respond to demands for the definition of law in terms of

factual correspondences fails to account for 'the idea of a rule, without which we cannot hope to elucidate even the most elementary forms of law' (78). And, says Hart, we cannot claim to make adequate statements about the existence of a rule in terms of habit. (Neither Austin nor any other thinker Hart takes to task does this, but we must let that pass.) The idea of a habit relates to observable uniformities of behaviour. Following a rule may to an outsider look like a habit. If a group has a rule requiring its members to meet in a bar every Saturday night, then such a gathering of its members could look like a habit and even take on elements of a habit. Yet it would always remain more than a habit. A habit would not oblige people to come nor would departing from the habit be a cause for criticism, much less a good reason for criticism. Nor does a rule correspond to a command, to orders that are backed by threats. We do not describe an order given by a gunman in a hold-up in the same terms as we describe a legal rule. For a start, not all legal rules require people to do or not to do something on pain of some harm that could result from not complying. Some rules enable people to do things. They enable people to make wills, they enable judges to judge, and so on. But even where the legal rule is a requirement backed by a sanction, it cannot be seen as 'the gunman situation writ large' (7). The immediate and transitory nature of the gunman's order does not, for example, accommodate the continuity of legal rules or the sustained commitments people have to rules in terms of rights and obligations.

With Hart, a conception of law in such terms as habits and commands would be confined to the 'external aspect' provided by an outside observer.

> For such an observer, deviations by a member of the group from normal conduct will be a sign that hostile reaction is likely to follow, and nothing more. His view will be like the view of one who, having observed the working of a traffic signal in a busy street for some time, limits himself to saying that when the light turns red there is a high probability that the traffic will stop. He treats the light merely as a natural *sign that* people will behave in certain ways, as clouds are a *sign that* rain will come. In so doing he will miss out a whole dimension of the social life of those whom he is watching, since for them the red light is not merely a sign that others

will stop: they look upon it as a *signal for* them to stop, and so a reason for stopping in conformity to rules which make stopping when the light is red a standard of behaviour and an obligation. To mention this is to bring into account the way in which the group regards its own behaviour. It is to refer to the internal aspect of rules seen from their internal point of view.

(87–8 – his emphasis)

It is this internal aspect which best encapsulates Hart's criticisms of the external conceptions of law (88). This aspect, to borrow Mac-Cormick's influential assessment, is 'the most distinctive and valuable element in Hart's work as a jurist' (1981: 29). Ironically it is the same internal aspect that undermines Hart's conceptions of law and legal system, as we shall see. I should now look at it in a little more detail.

Drawing on the idiom of linguistic philosophy, Hart locates the internal aspect of rule in contexts where rules operate and in the use people make of rules. Looking at such a use and such a context is a very different operation to the search for supposed correspondences to a rule that the external examiner is limited to. The external description of people's behaviour at traffic lights 'cannot be in terms of rules at all' (87). This is, admittedly, an 'extreme external point of view and does not give any account of the manner in which members of the group who accept the rules view their own regular behaviour' (87). But even the non-extreme observer 'who records *ab extra* the fact that a social group accepts such rules but does not himself accept them' has an external point of view, one which contrasts with the 'attitude of shared acceptance of rules' (99):

> What the external point of view . . . cannot reproduce is the way in which the rules function as rules in the lives of those who normally are the majority of society. These are the officials, lawyers, or private persons who use them, in one situation after another, as guides to the conduct of social life, as the basis for claims, demands, admissions, criticism, or punishment, viz., in all the familiar transactions of life according to rules.
>
> (88)

Yet again in the idiom of linguistic philosophy, Hart often resorts to games in order to make his point. His preferences are for chess and cricket:

Chess players do not merely have similar habits of moving the Queen in the same way which an external observer, who knew nothing about their attitude to the moves which they make, could record. In addition, they have a reflective critical attitude to this pattern of behaviour: they regard it as a standard for all who play the game. Each not only moves the Queen in a certain way himself but 'has views' about the propriety of all moving the Queen in that way. These views are manifested in the criticism of others and demands for conformity made upon others when deviation is actual or threatened, and in the acknowledgement of the legitimacy of such criticism and demands when received from others.

(55–6)

The external observer, or at least the extreme external observer, would not be able to 'distinguish, as compliance with an accepted rule, the adult chess-player's move from the action of the baby who merely pushed the piece into the right place' (137). The external observer does not act in relation to the rules 'as a member of the group which accepts and uses them as guides to conduct' (86). So we find that those following rules as guides to conduct, those living the rules, make statements in terms of someone being 'out' in a game of cricket, in terms of what 'must', 'should' or 'ought' to be done, in terms of 'having an obligation' and in terms of some action being 'wrong' (9, 56, 84). Such participants adopt 'a critical reflective attitude to certain patterns of behaviour as a common standard', 'as a general standard to be followed by the group as a whole', or 'as standards for the appraisal of their own and others' behaviour' (55–6, 96). Deviation from the standard, from a rule, 'is generally accepted as a *good reason*' for criticism or for some other 'hostile' reaction (54, 88 – Hart's emphasis). Or where 'our behaviour is challenged we are disposed to justify it by reference to the rule' (136; cf. Baker and Hacker 1985: 155, 159).

'There is some obscurity', says Harris, 'as to what . . . the concept of internal point of view stands for' (1980: 108). The question has become one of fervent jurisprudential debate in which 'internal' is conceived as internal to the person following the rule. But this line of enquiry is comprehensively frustrated by Hart. The internal aspect or point of view, he says, cannot be equated with approval of or moral support for the rule, nor with feelings of pressure or compulsion to follow it, nor with 'beliefs, fears and motives', nor indeed with mental experience at all (56, 81, 86, 198–9, 243). To ask what the element of the internal 'stands for', to seek correspondences to it in terms of mental processes, is to ignore Hart's whole orientation in linguistic philosophy. I will not go over the ground again except to say that the subtlety and diversity of use and context which Hart draws on in identifying the internal aspect are lost by reducing them in terms of mental processes (see e.g. Wittgenstein 1968: paras. 303–4). What such a reduction misses in particular is the social dimension of the internal aspect of rules. Hart constantly identifies the internal aspect in terms of 'demands for conformity made upon others', of a 'standard to be followed by the group as a whole', of 'a social group [which] accepts' the rules 'and uses them as guides to conduct' (55–6, 86, 99). The acceptance of the rule is manifested in such use (99). For 'the subtle kind of positivism' that is linguistic philosophy this use and the capabilities involved in it comprise the factual correspondences to the internal aspect (Pears 1971: 104, 172). As these points about the social dimension are crucial for the rest of my analysis of *The Concept of Law*, I will consider them a little more extensively.

Hart has a strange footnote supporting his conception of the internal aspect of rules. He simply refers to two works for 'similar views' to his own (242). The first is Winch, *The Idea of a Social Science and its Relation to Philosophy* (1958). Hart's internal aspect closely corresponds to ideas of Winch which closely correspond to those of Wittgenstein. The second work is Piddington, 'Malinowski's Theory of Needs' (1957), a work which would stand almost completely opposed to Winch's. But there is one significant area of agreement which these works share. For Winch, a rule is a standard reflectively applied and this is an essentially human activity. An animal cannot reflectively apply a rule. It acts out of ingrained habit (Winch 1958: 57–60). For Piddington, culture entails the resort to 'normative standards or values . . . crystallized in a system of symbols which enables individuals to evaluate the behaviour of others, irrespective of whether they are or are not themselves affected or involved'; and culture is distinctive of 'man's life as a social animal', something which does not characterize the lives of other animals (1957: 36–8). So also for Hart, unless we take account of the internal aspect of rules 'we cannot properly understand the whole distinctive style of human thought, speech, and action which is involved in the existence of rules and which constitutes the normative structure of society' (86). This all involves certain human skills and capacities (see e.g. 120). It involves understanding a rule as well as the calculation, organization and other techniques used in following a rule (Baker and Hacker 1985: 155, 159–63). Whether or not Wittgenstein would see all this as exclusively human, he did regard human behaviour as separable from animal behaviour and as characterized by the following of rules (Wittgenstein 1968: para. 25). Even 'if a lion could talk, we could not understand him', speaking, as he would, internally from within his distinct form of life (Wittgenstein 1968: 223). I will return to the internal aspect of rules when testing Hart's mythic 'foundations of a legal system'.

Hart now begins to introduce, beside the internal aspect, another requirement for the existence of legal rules: they must be somehow involved with officials. The origin of this requirement in Hart's account, apart from mere invocation, has puzzled acute observers (e.g. Moles 1987: 90–1). Hart does 'suppose' a legislator, Rex, and his successors, and '[i]n explaining the continuity of law-making power through a changing succession of individual legislators, it is natural to use the expressions "rule of succession", "title", "right to succeed", and "right to make law"' (51–3). What seems to be Hart's mode of argument here can be best approached through an example. Hart considers, as we saw, that these usages of 'right' and 'rule' cannot be accommodated by the Austinian notion of occasional and discontinuous commands or 'orders backed by threats'. Something better has to be found to sustain, for instance, the element of continuity involved in a rule and Hart locates this in the official world. But such a line of argument merely identifies a deficiency in one idea of law. It does not identify the official as the only way of making good the deficiency. The existence of Rex as the origin of the official world is merely given in Hart's original supposition and this was an invented example to aid presentation. Nor, it would seem, does Hart claim that an official element in 'right' and 'rule' is necessarily presupposed by the use of those terms. Despite Rex's fictional beginnings, Hart continues to insinuate Rex into his account until he is able to write of 'law-making, law-identifying and law-applying operations' being matters for 'the officials or experts of the system' as opposed to 'the mass of the population' or 'the ordinary citizen' which he now sees as ignorant and inadequate (59–60). Hart proceeds to secure this divide in a 'fabulous scene' with which we are by now familiar.

THE PRIMAL SCENE

This is the first step towards a 'fresh start' for jurisprudence (77). It is also a fresh start for Hart. Having relied integrally on linguistic philosophy and the creativity of language use to make his case, Hart now unceremoniously jettisons them and pursues a radically opposed perspective. He does, however, maintain a semblance of continuity by invoking a type of argument which has similarities to the mode that gave us Rex and the official world. As we saw, a view of law bearing an uncertain relation to that of Austin was found to be deficient because it did not accommodate 'the idea of a rule, without which we cannot hope to elucidate even the most elementary forms of law' (78). Now the slippage occurs. From the conclusion that a conception of law must include the idea of a rule, Hart moves towards confining law to rules. Rules provide 'the elements of law' and the foundations of a legal system (89, 97). The vaunted union of primary and secondary rules – the 'fresh start' which we consider shortly – is 'the heart of' or is 'at the centre of a legal system' (95–6). Such a 'union may be justly regarded as the "essence" of law' (151). Those distancing quotes around 'essence' as well as the relating of law to rules in foundational and biological metaphors – common preludes to modern myth – do perhaps evidence a residual reluctance simply to equate law with rules. This reluctance is an attenuated tribute to Hart's previous reliance on linguistic philosophy. As a linguistic philosopher, Hart would not seek the essence of law. He would not seek out what it is since for linguistic philosophy and for Hart that was a misconceived quest, as we saw. But it is a quest on which Hart now embarks. He founds the quest on the arbitrary and continuous reduction of law to a matter of rules (see also Hart 1987: 37–8). And he simply asserts that for the existence of such rules we need only look to other rules, for it is 'a very familiar chain of reasoning' that '[i]f the question is raised whether some suggested rule is legally valid, we must in order to answer the question use a criterion of validity provided by some other rule' (103). This stunning familiarity and Hart's confining of 'law' to rules, controversial as they have proved in Western jurisprudence, would be spectacularly alien to other major legal systems (see Geertz 1983: chapter 8). So much for the claimed universality of Hart's concept of law.

Nonetheless Hart confidently locates his fresh start for jurisprudence in a speculative universal history of early humanity. There Hart is witness to a primal scene in which law as the union of primary and secondary rules is conceived. This is the mythic return to origins, to what gives law form and makes it real. Spurious 'historical' origins create and give way to law's validating, formal origins. The myth of origin begins with a type of 'simple tribal society', 'a small community closely knit by ties of kinship, common sentiment, and belief and placed in a stable environment' (59, 89). The narration continues in a manner almost indistinguishable from Locke's account of law's creation which we encountered in chapter 4 (Locke 1965: 396 – paras. 124–6). The society is found to have only primary rules of obligation whereby 'human beings are required to do or abstain from certain actions, whether they wish to or not' (78–9). The primary rules are in Hart's view similar to custom. The imperative of social control means that they 'are in fact always found in primitive societies' where they have to be widely accepted in their internal aspect in order to be effective (89). Societies with only primary rules eventually appreciate the inadequacies of such an adamic simplicity and thus provide Hart with the components of his concept of law. In that state there would be no way of settling 'what the [primary] rules are or . . . the precise scope of some given rule' (90). The resulting uncertainty is cured by a rule of recognition providing 'conclusive identification of primary rules' in some authoritative, written form (92). Again, 'there will be no means, in such a society, of deliberately adapting the rules to changing circumstances, either by eliminating old rules or introducing new ones' (90). The resulting '*static* quality of the regime of primary rules' is cured by the introduction of 'rules of change' empowering 'an individual or body of persons to introduce new primary rules . . . and to eliminate old rules' (93 – his emphasis). Finally, there would be 'the *inefficiency* of the diffuse social pressures by which the rules are maintained' which would be cured by 'rules of adjudication . . . identifying the individuals who are to adjudicate' and identifying 'the procedure to be followed' (91, 94 – his emphasis).

> [T]he remedy for each defect might, in itself, be considered a step from the pre-legal into the legal world; since each remedy brings with it many elements that permeate law: certainly all three remedies together are enough to convert the regime of primary rules into what is indisputably a legal

193

system . . . . If we stand back and consider the structure which has resulted from the combination of primary rules of obligation with the secondary rules of recognition, change and adjudication, it is plain that we have here not only the heart of a legal system, but a most powerful tool for the analysis of much that has puzzled both the jurist and the political theorist.

(91, 95)

Whatever else this antique story may be, it is not linguistic philosophy. It is for a start an elaboration of Hart's arbitrary and essentialist confining of law to rules. But Hart's retreat from linguistic philosophy goes much further. Like those whom he has castigated for doing so, Hart now looks explicitly for what law is, not to its use and context. The discovery of law as the civilized outgrowth of the primal scene provides its essence. The very history forming law's essence supersedes itself and nullifies any continuing influence it could have. The pure, mechanical essence of law stands solitarily and autonomously apart from the forces that created it and apart from any informing context. If we explore the sources of what Hart is looking to, if we explore the knowledge that enables Hart to present this 'step from the pre-legal into the legal world' (244), we may more extensively grasp the mythic elevation of an essential law.

Hart's acknowledged source derives from the social anthropology of the twentieth century. Although he veers between the assertion that some if 'few' societies have existed without secondary rules and the assertion that such a state was 'never perhaps fully realized in any actual community', Hart does rely on anthropological 'studies of the nearest approximations to this state' (90, 244). Like much legal anthropology, these studies are concerned with the existence of so-called law in so-called primitive or savage societies. They share with Hart the technique of bringing a pre-existing conception of law to bear on the world, a conception corresponding to a type of Occidental law. The world then obliges by confirming that this idea of law is universally real. Anthropology has often provided tales of transition not unlike Hart's, tales of the development of societies from a primitive state and tales of the distinctive genesis of law in this development when public or official organization emerges out of diffuse and pervasive social norms (e.g. Hoebel 1954; Newman 1983).

194

Origins for such tales can also be found in Hart's second source, the evolutionary history of the nineteenth century. This source is not explicitly invoked but it pervades Hart's account. The evolutionary history of law is essentialist in that it requires 'the conceptual establishment of an entity [law in our case] that is progressing or evolving' (Bock 1979: 71). With this way of thinking, the entity is sustained despite the process of change by presenting transition as a step from one state containing the entity to another. The overall transition is always one from the simple to the complex, from the unified to the diverse. Impelled by this transition, the entity becomes increasingly distinct and differentiated but differentiation is always accompanied by a continued social integration, by an encompassing order in which the part of law is heightened. The entity in evolving responds to and overcomes the inadequacies of its prior form. It is conceptually viewed in its latest achieved stage and its universal history is told from that vantage point, a telling of how the entity came to be as it is. The parallels between this sort of story and Hart's account need not be laboured. Hart's mythic society at first has only primary rules which are 'a primitive or a rudimentary form of law' and which 'we are accustomed to contrast with a developed legal system' (84, 209). So Hart discerns, sometimes explicitly 'in the history of law' or 'as a matter of history', that societies have 'seen the advantages' of changing to more complex forms, that they have 'progressed to the point where' law and morality 'are distinguished as different forms of social control', and that with the introduction of secondary rules they 'step' from primitive or rudimentary law into a fully 'legal world', 'a step forward as important to society as the invention of the wheel' (41, 91–2, 95, 118). But with that step the creativity of the mass of society is exhausted and the legal dynamic is thereafter confined to the ranks of officials.

In the final and closest sources for Hart's story of the primal scene, we find him searching for 'the elements of law'(89), implicitly accompanying the philosophers of Enlightenment who sought the elements of forms in their origins. As we saw, numerous stories of Enlightenment not dissimilar to Hart's tell of life in a state of nature or in such variants as the savage state or a state regulated by custom. Law as intrinsic to (Western) civilization is contrasted constitutively with the state of nature. Law has its origins in the negation of the state of nature, its elements being a response to the inadequacies of that state. Even Hart's vaunted discovery of the elements of law as the union of primary and secondary rules is no more novel in this context than it was in the anthropological: the mythic origins of law in the tales of Enlightenment have it emerging when an official dimension operates on the state of nature, when a determining or 'positive' law is separated from and brought to bear on the 'negative . . . state which is styled a state of nature', to borrow the terms from Austin's version (1861–3: 122, 124).

As with Hart's story, in the thought of Enlightenment to account for origins is to establish enduring essence. The correspondence of origin and essence seems to be so obvious in Hart's account as not to require any explanation. Even in the speculative history that Hart offers, should there not be an appreciation that things change, that they can become radically different to what they were? But despite its mode of presentation, this is not an enquiry into history or into any known state of affairs. Hart, as we saw, is inconsistent on the issue of whether there ever was a society which had only primary rules. Yet such a society is his starting point and the inadequacy of having only primary rules provides the seemingly historical impetus for his elements of law. But uncertainties and absences of evidence were, as we saw in chapter 3, no restraint on the thought of Enlightenment. Answers can be found elsewhere. Using Hart's terms for aspects of his primal scene, the answer is 'discoverable by reason' or in 'natural necessity', in 'truisms about human nature', in 'elementary truths concerning human beings' (89, 189, 195). In the Enlightenment, a transcendent subjectivity and ordering reason produced constant elements that underlie the apparent changes and diversity of an entity and provided the common ground unifying and integrating it. So Hart's elements of law provide what is common and constant in the diversity of law's manifestations. Given the constant character of these elements, an enquiry into origins will reveal them as they are now, and reveal them more readily because in origins we find the elements in their simple forms before the addition of complex and obscuring shapes. Finally, the concern with constant elements in the thought of Enlightenment was a concern with the necessary order of things, with harmony and equilibrium. This concern transfers in Hart's turn to a cohering 'control' as integral to society and law (89, 191). Law is a result of imperatives of order and itself orders. It is *ordo ordinans*, ordering order (cf. Cassirer 1955: 240).

Thus, if we 'stand back' and consider Hart's story of the primal scene enlightened by its three sources, we do not find a diversity of ideas of 'law' emerging from its various uses and contexts. Hart seeks and finds elements that constitute a singular and constant essence of law. This essence comes from a Western conception of law, the terms of which inhabit and shape the whole enquiry. Understandably enough, those terms are readily discovered in the enquiry and emerge reinforced from it. In these terms law, whilst being intrinsic to social order, acts on and controls society. It does this determinatively through official performances which emanate from a vantage point of distinct domination, one necessarily separated from the society that is ordered and controlled. All of which bespeaks a peculiar 'western cosmology' (Strathern 1985: 128), not a universal history of law as Hart would have it.

At this stage, then, we have two opposed Harts – the linguistic philosopher and the enunciator of law's essence. And we have two opposing sets of consequences of this division. With one, we have popular usages, an internal aspect of rules and active, reflective subjects, all of which are at the very core of Hart's initial analysis. With the other, there is the dominance of official determinations, a dominance finally emerging as universal necessity in that natural history of law which Hart finds in the primal scene. It is at this point of cavernous difference that Hart presents a concluded, resolved picture in 'the foundations of a legal system', the 'buckle' holding together 'the whole of his normative legal theory' (Cotterell 1989: 100).

THE APOTHEOSIS OF THE OFFICIAL

These foundations of a legal system mark the triumph of one side of the duality – that is, the triumph of official determinations. The other side of the duality is reduced by Hart in terms of rules and their internal aspect. Hart effects the triumph of official determinations by making the internal aspect necessary only for them. Such a resolution is reached through an astonishing compression of contradictions. Having based both his criticism of previous ideas of law and the lineaments of his alternative on the necessity for rules to have an internal aspect, Hart proceeds to deny that necessity. Having said that the internal aspect cannot be envisaged in terms of individual mental states, he now proceeds to treat of its presence and absence in terms of individual mental states. And having thus subordinated the internal aspect to individual mentality, Hart posits the possibility of a society in which that mentality eliminates the internal aspect for 'the ordinary citizen'. This is a strange society. It is a society without social relations, a society which Hart bolsters with desperate metaphor rather than sociolinguistic or sociological observation. It is a society which lacks attributes which Hart elsewhere in *The Concept of Law* considers necessary for the existence of any society. And the contradictions multiply. Again myth is evoked to mediate them.

I will now provide a more extensive guide to these contradictions after outlining the so-called foundations of the legal system. There are for Hart:

> two minimum conditions necessary and sufficient for the existence of a legal system. On the one hand those rules of behaviour which are valid according to the system's ultimate criteria of validity must be generally obeyed, and, on the other hand, its rules of recognition specifying the criteria of legal validity and its rules of change and adjudication must be effectively accepted as common public standards of official behaviour by its officials. The first condition is the only one which private citizens *need* satisfy: they may obey each 'for his part only' and from any motive whatever; though in a healthy society they will in fact often accept these rules as common standards of behaviour and acknowledge an obligation to obey them.
>
> (113 – his emphasis)

For 'the ordinary citizen' to have this 'merely personal concern with rules':

> He need not think of his conforming behaviour as 'right', 'correct', or 'obligatory'. His attitude, in other words, need not have any of that critical character which is involved whenever social rules are accepted and types of conduct are treated as general standards. He need not, though he may, share the internal point of view accepting the rules as standards for all to whom they apply. Instead, he may think of the rule only as something demanding action from *him* under threat of penalty.
>
> (112 – his emphasis)

I will look first at what this account does to that internal aspect of rules which I considered in detail earlier. We saw that for Hart the operation of legal rules necessarily involved an internal aspect. This is entailed in people's '*use* [of] the rules as standards for the appraisal of their own and others' behaviour' (96 – his emphasis). The internal aspect has an integral social dimension. Not only do people use rules to evaluate the conduct of others as well as their own but along with Hart we must conceive of the internal aspect in terms of the social group accepting the rules, in terms of 'the way in which the group regards its own behaviour' (88, 99). The internal aspect is inseparable from 'the whole distinctive style of human thought, speech, and action which is involved in the existence of rules and which constitutes the normative structure of society' (86). So, for the internal aspect individual 'beliefs, fears and motives' are irrelevant (81). It is not tied to individual attitudes to a rule. 'Hence there is no contradiction in saying of some hardened swindler, and it may often be true, that he had an obligation to pay the rent but felt no pressure to pay when he made off without doing so' (86).

In terms of Hart's analysis thus far and in terms of linguistic philosophy these individual mentalities and the internal aspect are incommensurable, but we now reach a point which takes Hart almost as far from his origins in linguistic philosophy as it is possible to go. For he now treats the internal aspect not only as commensurable with but as subordinated to individual mentalities. A person can now follow a rule but opt out of the internal aspect simply by adopting an appropriate mental state. Even if we granted what Hart calls this 'merely personal concern with the rules', such a concern cannot extend to the evaluation of the conduct of others in terms of the internal aspect (112). The person who obeys 'for his part only' does not thereby create a ruleless world. Sadists for example might not accept a rule prohibiting assault as long as they conceive of themselves doing the assaulting. But for their own security and social life they could not be indifferent on this score to the rule-orientation of others. It would be impossible to go into society without using the rules to evaluate the behaviour of others – to 'walk among men as if before lions' (see Riley 1986: 165). It is impossible, in short, to ignore 'the normative structure of society' (86). Yet just such indifference and ignorance would have to typify Hart's always singular person or citizen who always in the singular 'obeys for his part only'.

There are a few other points which amplify the incongruence of Hart's position. For one, we may ask what could relate these very 'private citizens' to each other, relate all the citizen isolates who 'obey each "for his part only"' (113). They would have no social bonds. Hart confines them tightly in terms of fear and inertia and has them relating solely and passively to the dictates of officials (112). If they were sentient at all this inertia would have to be complete since there would be no basis on which these citizen isolates could overcome inertia and relate to each other. So perhaps they have no relevant or significant sentience. If they do not partake of the internal aspect, perhaps they adopt the external aspect of the outside observer. But they cannot because they are not outside observers and Hart would only go so far on this score as to say that the 'external point of view may very nearly reproduce the way in which the rules function in the lives of certain members of the group, namely those who reject its rules and are only concerned with them when and because they judge that unpleasant consequences are likely to follow violation' (88). If neither the external nor the internal aspect is involved in following a rule in such terms, then what is? Hart's ultimate answer seems to be no aspect at all. For a society made up of such people would be 'deplorably sheeplike' and 'the sheep might end up in the slaughter-house' (114). Such a deplorably tired metaphor is apt in that Hart does see the internal aspect of rules as 'distinctive . . . of human thought, speech and action' (86). But how would such an in-human society operate? What exact mechanisms of stimulus-response, what minutely regulated but inexorable appetites, would take the place of the critical, reflective human that Hart previously saw as intrinsic to the following of legal rules? Hart does not pursue the point. It stands opposed to much else in his book. It stands opposed to his assertion of humanity as integral to the following of rules. It stands opposed to his extensive criticism of other theorists for 'treating all rules as directives only to officials' since this does not take account of the active and reflective ways 'in which these are spoken of, thought of, and actually used in social life' (78). It stands opposed to a need if law is to exist for 'multitudes of individuals' to be able to understand conduct required of them as it is prescribed in general rules (121). And it stands opposed to his finding a minimum content of law involved in the very existence of society, a minimum content whereby people have to relate to each other in 'mutual forbearance and compromise', have to 'co-operate' and have to make and sustain promises (189–93) – all of which entails an internal aspect of rules widely disseminated in society.

But why, ultimately, this unpropitious resort to the society of sheep? In attacking existing positivist theories of various kinds, Hart located an internal aspect of rules and in this he endowed the populace with a critical reflective attitude, with abilities to act on and to evaluate standards of behaviour, with the capacity to pursue a highly skilled enterprise (see Hirst and Jones 1987: 29; also Baker and Hacker 1985: 155–63). The boar had been released into the vineyard. If the orthodoxy of legal positivism and law's autonomy are to be sustained, the populace has to be relegated, in the last instance as it were, to its inert state. The official emerges whole and impregnable to determine, to posit that which all others must obey. Introduced with the insidious supposition of Rex and his successors, then rendered inevitable by that natural history of the primal scene, the official now becomes the apotheosis of the legal, the only necessarily sentient element in law and hence the only source of the legally positive. Hart thus effects the separation of the rule from its use and enables it to be treated definitively as so separated. His project culminates in a simple, a very simple, claim to authority. As in the colonial situation, this authority of the official is supreme, coming from outside society and acting upon it. Use and context and the diversity of uses and contexts are ignored. As Césaire says, the rule of the European bourgeoisie has torn up the root of diversity (Césaire 1955: 69–70).

In this deracination of rules the realm of the official is an assumption of pure and complete authority that transcends and determines use and context. We can appreciate this by returning to the disparaged Austin. Hart's 'two minimum conditions necessary and sufficient for the existence of a legal system' are mocked in their correspondence to Austin's idea of law as expounded in *The Province of Jurisprudence Determined*: 'The matter of jurisprudence is positive law: law, simply and strictly so called: or law set by political superiors to political inferiors,' by superiors to whom 'habitual obedience must be rendered by the *generality* or *bulk* of . . . members' of a political society (1861–3: 1, 174 – I – his emphasis). Although, for Hart, the only 'need' of official authority is obedience from 'private citizens', yet 'in a healthy society' these citizens will 'often accept' the rules produced by officials and not simply obey them (112–13). But even this salubrious whimper has no necessary part in a legal system. Hart, in the end, grounds his scheme on an unlimited and unified authority whose basis is never explicitly asserted, apart from its origin in a primal scene

Sampford 1989: 35–6, 44–6). He is squarely in the tradition of Hobbes and Austin with their foundational reliance on the savage state.

The otherwise improbable connection between the primal scene and our present legal condition is secured in myth. The primal scene is, in terms of Occidental mythology, the point of origin from the negation of which creation issues forth. It exists in a time of beginnings, of absolute truths whose empirical authenticities cannot be tested. It is, like Trobriand myth, 'beyond fact, beyond reason and refers to events beyond memory and ordinary time' (Cohen 1969: 344). It provides both the foundation of law and, what is massively implicit in Hart's account, the continuing force which gives law 'effectiveness and duration' (Eliade 1965: 11). In Hart's story, there is a standard mythic transformation from *prima materia*, primal matter, into the plane of culture – a 'breakthrough' that establishes the entity (Eliade 1963: 6). From the initial, the natural and the raw emerges the differentiated form, set apart from yet sharing in what has made it. The process of creating and sustaining the entity is often mediated in myth through figures that straddle the realms of transcendent creation and its mundane outcome. One of the instances we met was Adam who, with his naming inventory and ordained organizing, was the first official.

This placing of Hart's concept of law within the European mythology of origin can help explain the silent suppression of linguistic philosophy along with the popular creation of meaning. All the inhabitants of the primal scene, from the savages of North America to the colonized of Africa, shared a convenient characteristic which prevented their contributing to linguistic use: they could not speak and thus had to be spoken for. In the imperial mentality which informs Hart's account and its sources, true knowledge is brought by the European to the mute and inglorious savages. Their reality is thereby known for the first time – known properly and fully both in itself and in the universal nature of things. Inadequate local knowledges are infinitely encompassed and given adequacy by European knowledge which is, in turn, elevated in its relation to them. Being without a history or a project of their own, the savages and the colonized take their uniform characteristics from the uniform European perception of them. This provides the common ground, the unassailable objectivity, founding the mythic universal history of 'early man', a history beyond which only some have progressed. The imperial cast of mind, as Rackett perceives it, neutralized myriad existences and meanings into a crude, mythical uniformity 'where "whiteness" signifies positivity, identity and certitude, and "blackness" signifies negativity, difference and transgression' (Rackett 1985: 195).

To draw out the closer connections between Hart's conception of law and this mythology I will return to the colonial situation (see also Skillen 1977: 102–7). The stock delusions attending colonial rule permeate Hart's story. Native society is simple, small and self-contained. It is characterized by uncertainty, stasis, ineffici-ency, and by a lawless or only incipiently legal condition. The colonists claim to bring a civilization which will provide many things, among them security and order, incorporation within a dynamic history, efficiency, law, and the opportunity for progress by means of social functions becoming differentiated. The natives long for all this in the depth of their being, long for it as their own completion. As the colonial situation presents an administered reality, it is the official who is to bring to fruition the incipient humanity of the native.

There are some less obtrusive if equally potent dimensions to Hart's repertoire of myth. For one, he simply adopts the law of a 'country', 'municipal legal systems' and 'municipal law in a modern state' as paradigm (3, 7, 77). These categories are freigh-ted with the mythic power of the nation in its identifying of a people and their law, something we explored in chapter 4. It was the mediation of the superior nations, or comity of superior nations, that gave mythic credence to claims like Hart's that the law of the Occident was universal. Law, in its turn, serves to elevate national identity in opposition to the particular and in orientation towards the universal. The nation shares mythic themes with Hart's insinuated king whom we met more recently. As well as inserting the idea of official authority into his story, Rex serves a more traditional mythic purpose for Hart as a vehicle of law's continuity. 'King is a name of Continuance', in the words of a sixteenth-century case, 'The King never dies' (see Goodrich and Hachamovitch 1991: 170). There may even be connections be-tween Hart's 'fresh start' for law and the introduction of Rex since in many mythologies coronation is a 'new birth' of society (Hocart 1927: 189–90).

The monarch and the nation are creative forms of the powerful symbolism of the centre. Hart's explicit equivalent is an ultimate rule of recognition, a rule on which the unity, coherence and very existence of a legal system depends. That is, any legal system is supposedly made up of rules and the legal existence or validity of a rule is supposedly determined by reference to another rule superior to it in a hierarchy until an ultimate rule of recognition is reached. The existence of that rule, in turn, depends on its being accepted in practice by the officials it has presumably created. It is audacious enough to take a contentious description of one legal system and to elevate it mythically to a universal prescription, but in doing this Hart takes to the extreme the most spectacular juris-prudential borrowing from myth, the 'sources thesis' (see e.g. Raz 1980: 210–16). A law takes existence and validity simply from its source or, in standard mythic terms, from its origin. To know the source of the thing is to know its essence – the contrast with linguistic philosophy could hardly be more stark – and in myth the force of origin is also a force of continuing creation. A law con-tinues as a source of other laws or as a source of effectiveness and validity for legal relations. The rule of recognition is the ultimate concentration of the mythic dynamic disseminated throughout law whereby reality or validity is found in an infinitely repeatable return to origins.

Myth even mediates contradiction between Hart's initial use of linguistic philosophy and his resort to essence and authority. The mythic legal subject we encountered in chapter 4 precisely matches and combines the elements in contradiction. This sub-ject, like the figure of the individual at the centre of modern mythology, is an infinitely responsive being. The subject is also enormously skilled at integrating an enormous range of influences and determinations and bringing them to bear on itself. In this, the subject is not simply an abject receptacle but a reflective and effective being, participating efficiently in its own subjection. People inhabiting Hart's legal system are similar beings. With their internal perspective on rules, they are endowed with large skills and capacities. They are participants and players, existentially and socially committed to a 'form of life' identified in the vibrant terms of language (cf. Wittgenstein 1968: paras. 19, 23, 241). In their relation to law they do not simply accept or obey an immediate imperative. They have the law and they live the law. But like custom and other popular indwellings we have encountered, this element in law becomes marginalized in the face of authority. The only necessary attitude for the 'subject' then becomes an acceptant or quiescent one. Hart's essential model becomes the sheep. This is the most extreme rendering possible of that other side of legal subjectivity described in chapter 4, the subject's self-contraction in a solitary, apprehensive and yet unavoidable involvement with what cannot be known or fully known. But this does not result in any diminishing or qualification of the subject's relation to law. It is a full, and fully responsive allegiance. 'We are', says Dworkin as mythmaker, 'subjects of law's empire, liegemen to its methods and ideals, bound in spirit while we debate what we must therefore do' (Dworkin 1986: vii).

This forlorn captive is found, I think, in Kafka's parable of being 'before the law' (1988b: 161–2). 'A man from the country', coming perhaps from a natural community, 'begs for admittance to the Law'. He begs to the official door-keeper, the first in a hierarchy of keepers who assert exclusive power over entry to the law. This door-keeper refuses immediate entrance through the open door-way to the law but he does not rule out the possibility of later entry. After a lifetime of waiting by the door and of seeking to persuade the official to let him enter, the man from the country is near death, 'all that he has experienced during the whole time of his sojourn condenses in his mind into one question'. He says to the door-keeper:

> 'Everyone strives to attain the Law . . . how does it come about, then, that in all these years no one has come seeking admittance but me?' The door-keeper perceives that the man is at the end of his strength and his hearing is failing, so he bellows in his ear: 'No one but you could gain admittance through this door, since this door was intended only for you. I am now going to shut it.'
>
> (Kafka 1988b: 162)

With that the parable ends and the multitude of interpretations begins, starting with the debate in Kafka's text (1988b: 163–7). The contrary yet co-existing dimensions of legal subjectivity are encapsulated at the outset of the debate:

> The story contains two important statements made by the door-keeper about admission to the Law, one at the begin-ning, the other at the end. The first statement is: that he cannot admit the man at the moment, and the other is: that this door was intended only for the man. If there were a contradiction between the two, you would be right and the

door-keeper would have deluded the man. But there is no contradiction. The first statement, on the contrary, even implies the second.

(Kafka 1988b: 163)

I will expand this interpretation a little by overlaying Hart's account on the parable. Only the official can properly recognize law and we relate to law definitively through the official. In that relation we exist apart from any assured knowledge of that which rules us. Yet we are operatively engaged in the law we are separated from and we necessarily share that engagement with others. The contradiction between separation and such an engagement is mediated in an acceptant subjectivity and in a purely personal destiny 'before the law' – 'this door was intended only for you' (Kafka 1988b: 162). We are kept ever attentive and always waiting outside the law but fixed to it. In this condition, we are and have to be 'really free': when the man from the country 'sits down on the stool by the side of the door and stays there for the rest of his life, he does it of his own free will; in the story there is no mention of any compulsion' (Kafka 1988b: 165).

MYTH AND CONCEPT

Having elevated authority, Hart now vainly seeks to subject it to law as rules having essential meanings – meanings as to which there can be 'no doubts' in 'the vast, central areas of the law' (149–50). As we saw, once Hart had simply asserted that law was a matter of rules he could in his fresh start found a concept of law and the elements of law in rules. But when he came to tie everything together in the foundations of the legal system, Hart discovered that law need only be a matter of official authority. This raises a problem since:

> Hart's legal theory portrays law as a self-regulating system of rules. The rule of recognition and the other secondary rules are seen as governing the entire process of production, inter-pretation, enforcement, amendment and repeal of rules within the legal system. In contrast to Austin's picture of a legal order as the expression and instrument of all-too-human political power (the power of the sovereign and its delegates), Hart's image of law is that of a system in which rules govern power-holders; in which rules, rather than

people, govern. What is, indeed, implied here is an aspect of
the deeply resonant political symbol so obviously missing
from Austin's jurisprudence – the symbol of the Rule of Law,
a 'government of laws and not of men'.

(Cotterrell 1989: 99)

Hence the resort to essential meaning. Hart would not go so far as
to say that legal rules are always clear and have just to be applied.
But for rules to be uncertain and simply subject to human determination is for Hart a 'nightmare' (Hart 1983: chapter 4). Legal
rules, he is relieved to find, do have a persistent 'core' of certain
meaning but in practice there is also a 'penumbra' of uncertainty
where officials have discretion in applying them. What Hart is
saying here, astonishing as it may sound, is that in considering the
meaning of a rule there are 'paradigm, clear cases' at the core
where there are 'no doubts' (125, 149). Official discretion is confined to cases of penumbral uncertainty. That discretion presumably remains of the law because to characterize it 'would be to
characterize whatever is specific or peculiar in legal reasoning'
(124). Such cases of uncertainty are exceptional. In the result
there are 'wide areas of conduct which are successfully controlled
ab initio by rule', where determinate rules 'guide' officials (130,
132). In this the official merely draws out of the rule what is latent
within it (see Goodrich 1987: 56). Hart thus resorts to the very
mode of determining meaning, to 'the bewitchment . . . by means
of language' (Wittgenstein 1968: para. 109), which had plagued
jurisprudence heretofore and from which he was to liberate us.
The meaning of the rule is divorced from its use and context. It lies
within to be discerned in an essential, a paradigm core. This is the
concern with 'common qualities' which Hart considered so con-
fused and which is the exact antithesis of the perspective in which
he initially set his project (234; cf. Wittgenstein 1967: para. I–4,
1968: para. 50).

Hart's essentialist position is lent superficial plausibility by the
presence of some stability in the interpretation of some legal rules.
But this stability is not one that exists apart from officials or that
circumscribes their action from without. What is or is not 'clear'
for the time being is a product of official judgement. Apart from
drawing on what judges do in order to illustrate his argument,
Hart does not say how the core is to be distinguished from the
penumbra. Nor does he say how a clear meaning can be swept

aside by official judgement and replaced by a different meaning, as does happen. Fish puts the matter with characteristic cogency:

> The question is not whether there are in fact plain cases – there surely are – but, rather, of what is their plainness a condition and a property? Hart's answer must be that a plain case is inherently plain, plain in and of itself, plain independently of the interpretive activities it can then be said to direct. But it takes only a little reflection to see that the truth is exactly the reverse. A plain case is a case that was once *argued*: that is, its configurations were once in dispute; at a certain point one characterization of its meaning and significance – of its *rule* – was found to be more persuasive than its rivals; and at *that* point the case became settled, became perspicuous, became undoubted, became plain. Plainness, in short, is not a property of the case itself – there is no case itself – but of an interpretive history in the course of which one interpretive agenda . . . has subdued another. That history is then closed, but it can always be reopened.
>
> (Fish 1989: 523)

Or, in terms of linguistic philosophy, 'the rules do not provide a fixed point of reference, because they always allow divergent interpretations. What really gives the practices their stability is that we agree in our interpretations of the rules' (Pears 1971: 168). Simply, 'there is as much stability as there is' (Pears 1971: 168).

Essential stability is achieved in the mythic elevation of the concept which, in its dominating fixity, denies the fluidity and negotiability of legal rules. The concept is complete and 'fully manifested' (cf. Eliade 1968: 16). It is able repeatedly and eternally to evoke and apply its constant content, subsuming the diversity of instances to its uniform and exemplary rule. The concept is thus a condensation of the formative dynamic of myth (cf. Adorno and Horkheimer 1979: 12). In giving substance to law as legal rules, the concept enables law to rule and to remain set apart from contingency and temporality. Law, it would seem, is protected by 'the rigidity and exclusiveness which concepts were generally compelled to assume wherever language united the community of rulers with the giving of orders' (Adorno and Horkheimer 1979: 22). Austin's triumph would appear to be complete.

Hart's attempt to preserve law from an involving use and context fails, except as myth. I will mark that failure by eliminating the one elaborated example Hart gives of a legal rule with a core of certainty and a penumbra of doubt. For Hart the stakes here are high because the rule is that ultimate rule of recognition, founding the existence and coherence of the whole legal system. If there is no core of certainty to the ultimate rule, if it cannot be held inviolable, then this edifice is unsupported. But there seems to be no risk of this. The rule Hart chooses is impregnable. It contains 'the English doctrine of the sovereignty of Parliament', of which 'the formula "Whatever the Queen in Parliament enacts is law" is an adequate expression' (144–5). Integral to this rule is 'the principle that no earlier Parliament can preclude its "successors" from repealing its legislation' (145). A later statute will always override an inconsistent earlier one. The rule thus ensures the impossibility of its being dislodged. Add to this the view of Wade and Bradley in their text on constitutional law that 'this doctrine is to be found in all legal systems' (1985: 71) and Hart's position would seem assured.

Nonetheless, even for this rule, he says, 'doubts can arise as to its meaning or scope; we can ask what is meant by "enacted by Parliament"' (145). He then refers to instances where a legislature has changed what is called the manner and form in which legislation is constituted. Parliament may enact that a type of legislation could in future only be passed by a special majority or with the addition of another element such as a referendum. Would that enactment bind later parliaments or would it, on the contrary, be subject to later legislation inconsistent with it? This, says Hart, is a penumbral area of doubt. Changing the manner and form of legislation may bind future parliaments but:

> if this device were valid, Parliament could achieve by its use very much the same results as those which the accepted doctrine, that Parliament cannot bind its successors, seems to put beyond its power. For though, indeed, the difference between circumscribing the area over which Parliament can legislate, and merely changing the manner and form of legislation, is clear enough in some cases, in effect these categories shade into each other. A statute which, after fixing a minimum wage for engineers, provided that no bill concerning engineers' pay should have effect as law unless confirmed by resolution of the Engineers' Union and went on to entrench this provision, might indeed secure all that, in

practice, could be done by a statute which fixed the wage 'for ever', and then crudely prohibited its repeal altogether. Yet an argument, which lawyers would recognize as having some force, can be made to show that although the latter would be ineffective under the present rule of continuing parliamentary sovereignty, the former would not.

(147)

In other words, the core and the penumbra cannot be distinguished. Or rather, they can only be distinguished by a return to authority – by the mysterious invocation of a way 'which lawyers would recognize', by resort to 'whatever is specific or peculiar in legal reasoning' (124). Essence becomes the assertion of a particular use and context. This is simply 'the language of legal faith' (Goodrich 1987: chapter 3). It is also the language of ultimately unquestionable legal authority. Having started with a regenerative vision of truth as something 'we' share and create, Hart ends with the wearying reassertion of truth as something in which we can only acquiesce.

This is enough to dispose of the matter but I should add that the enduring core of the rule which Hart identifies has no existence even in the assertions of authority. As I have shown elsewhere, the community of lawyers in Britain, and even in England, is riven over the ultimate rule of recognition which Hart advances as foundational, sustaining and inviolate (Fitzpatrick 1991: 25). There are several competing rules of recognition. For Hart, such a situation marks 'the pathology of a legal system,' 'a sub-standard, abnormal case containing within it the threat that the legal system will dissolve' (114, 119). The pathology must be healed or a new, singular whole must take the place of the stricken entity. Yet fundamental irresolution has long been the standard, normal case of the 'legal system' of the so-called United Kingdom. There is neither an ultimate rule nor that settled official support for it essential to Hart's scheme. The last supports fall away and the sources of law's being disappear. Outside of myth, it has no existence.

BIBLIOGRAPHY

Adorno, T. and Horkheimer, M. (1979). *Dialectic of Enlightenment*, London: Verso.

Althusser, L. (1971). *Lenin and Philosophy and Other Essays*, London: New Left Books.

Althusser, L. (1972). *Politics and History: Montesquieu, Rousseau, Hegel and Marx*, London: New Left Books.

Anderson, P. (1974). *Lineages of the Absolutist State*, London: New Left Books.

Arthur, C. (1978). 'Editor's Introduction', in E. B. Pashukanis, *Law and Marxism: A General Theory*, London: Ink Links.

Arthurs, H. W. (1985). *'Without the Law': Administrative Justice and Legal Pluralism in Nineteenth-Century England*, Toronto: University of Toronto Press.

Auden, W. H. (1948). *The Age of Anxiety: A Baroque Eclogue*, London: Faber & Faber.

Auden, W. H. (1966). 'Law Like Love', in *Collected Shorter Poems 1927–1957*, London: Faber & Faber.

Austin, J. (1861–3). *The Province of Jurisprudence Determined*, 2nd edn and *Lectures on Jurisprudence*, 3 vols, London: John Murray.

Axtell, J. (1985). *The Invasion Within: The Conquest of Cultures in Colonial North America*, New York: Oxford University Press.

Baker, G. P. and Hacker, P. M. S. (1985). *Wittgenstein: Rules, Grammar and Necessity: An Analytical Commentary on the 'Philosophical Investigations': Volume 2*, Oxford: Basil Blackwell.

Balibar, E. (1990). 'Paradoxes of Universality', in D. T. Goldberg (ed.), *Anatomy of Racism*, Minneapolis: University of Minnesota Press.

Barker, M. (1981). *The New Racism: Conservatives and the Ideology of the Tribe*, London: Junction Books.

Barnes, J. (1990). *A History of the World in 10^1/2 Chapters*, London: Pan.

Barnett, H. A. and Yach, D. M. (1985). 'The Teaching of Jurisprudence and Legal Theory in British Universities and Polytechnics', *Legal Studies* 5: 151–7.

Barron, A. (1990). 'Legal Discourse and Colonization of the Self in the Modern State', in A. Carty (ed.), *Post-Modern Law: Enlightenment, Revolution and the Death of Man*, Edinburgh: Edinburgh University Press.

211

Barthes, R. (1973). *Mythologies*, St Albans: Paladin.

Becker, C. L. (1932). *The Heavenly City of the Eighteenth-Century Philosophers*, New Haven: Yale University Press.

Bentham, J. (1970a). *Of Laws in General*, London: Athlone Press.

Bentham, J. (1970b). *An Introduction to the Principles of Morals and Legislation*, London: Athlone Press.

Berman, H. J. (1983). *Law and Revolution: The Formation of the Western Legal Tradition*, Cambridge: Harvard University Press.

Bernal, M. (1987). *Black Athena: The Afroasiatic Roots of Classical Civilization, Volume I: The Fabrication of Ancient Greece 1785–1985*, London: Free Association Books.

Bidney, D. (1958). 'Myth, Symbolism and Truth', in T. A. Sebeok (ed.), *Myth: A Symposium*, Bloomington and London: Indiana University Press.

Black, D. (1976). *The Behaviour of Law*, New York: Academic Press.

Blackstone, W. (1825). *Commentaries on the Laws of England*, 16th edn, London: T. Cadell and J. Butterworth & Son.

Bloch, M. (1974). 'Symbols, Song, Dance and Features of Articulation: Is Religion an Extreme Form of Traditional Authority?', *European Archive of Sociology*, XV: 55–81.

Bloch, M. (1986). *From Blessing to Violence: History and Ideology in the Circumcision Ritual of the Merina of Madagascar*, Cambridge: Cambridge University Press.

Bloch, M. and Bloch, J. H. (1980). 'Women and the Dialectics of Nature in Eighteenth Century French Thought', in C. P. MacCormack and M. Strathern (eds), *Nature, Culture and Gender*, Cambridge: Cambridge University Press.

Bock, K. (1979). 'Theories of Progress, Development, Evolution', in T. Bottomore and R. Nisbet (eds), *A History of Sociological Analysis*, London: Heinemann.

Borges, J. L. (1970). *Labyrinths*, Harmondsworth: Penguin.

Bourdieu, P. (1988). *Homo Academicus*, Cambridge: Polity Press.

Bozeman, A. D. (1971). *The Future of Law in a Multicultural World*, Princeton: Princeton University Press.

Brantlinger, P. (1985). 'Victorians and Africans: The Genealogy of the Myth of the Dark Continent', *Critical Inquiry*, 12 (1): 166–203.

Broekman, J. M. (1986). 'Legal Subjectivity as a Precondition for the Intertwinement of Law and the Welfare State', in G. Teubner (ed.), *Dilemmas of Law in the Welfare State*, Berlin and New York: Walter de Gruyter.

Cain, M. (1986). 'Who Loses Out on Paradise Island? The Case of Defendant Debtors in County Court', in I. Ramsey (ed.), *Debtors and Creditors*, Abingdon: Professional Books.

Cain, M. (1988). 'Beyond Informal Justice', in R. Matthews (ed.), *Informal Justice?*, London: Sage.

Cain, M. and Hunt, A. (1979). *Marx and Engels on Law*, London and New York: Academic Press.

Carr, H. (1984). 'Woman/Indian: "The American" and His Others', in F. Barker *et al.* (eds), *Europe and its Others: Volume Two*, Colchester: University of Essex.

Carty, A. (1990). 'Introduction: Post-Modern Law', in A. Carty (ed.) *Post-Modern Law: Enlightenment Revolution and the Death of Man*, Edinburgh: Edinburgh University Press.

Carty, A. (1991). 'English Constitutional Law from a Postmodernist Perspective', in P. Fitzpatrick (ed.), *Dangerous Supplements: Resistance and Renewal in Jurisprudence*, London: Pluto Press; Durham: Duke University Press.

Cassirer, E. (1955). *The Philosophy of the Enlightenment*, Boston: Beacon Press.

Césaire, A. (1955). *Discours sur le Colonialisme*, Paris: Présence Africaine.

Chatterjee, P. (1986). *Nationalist Thought and the Colonial World: A Derivative Discourse?*, London: Zed Books.

Cohen, G. A. (1978). *Karl Marx's Theory of History: A Defence*, Oxford: Clarendon Press.

Cohen, P. S. (1969). 'Theories of Myth', *Man N.S.*, 4: 337–53.

Collis, R. J. M. (1966). 'Physical Health and Psychiatric Disorder in Nigeria', *Transactions of the American Philosophical Society, New Series*, 56 (4).

Condorcet, Marquis de (1965). 'The Progress of the Human Mind', in I. Schneider (ed.), *The Enlightenment: The Culture of the Eighteenth Century*, New York: George Braziller.

Connolly, W. E. (1988). *Political Theory and Modernity*, Oxford: Basil Blackwell.

Conrad, J. (1960). *Heart of Darkness* in *Three Short Novels*, New York: Bantam.

Cornford, F. M. (1932). *Before and After Socrates*, Cambridge: Cambridge University Press.

Cornford, F. M. (1957). *From Religion to Philosophy: A Study in the Origins of Western Speculation*, New York: Harper & Row.

Cotterrell, R. (1989). *The Politics of Jurisprudence: A Critical Introduction to Legal Philosophy*, London and Edinburgh: Butterworths.

Cottrell, A. (1984). *Social Classes in Marxist Theory*, London: Routledge & Kegan Paul.

Curtin, P. D. (1964). *The Image of Africa: British Ideas and Action, 1780–1964*, Madison: University of Wisconsin Press.

Curtin, P. D. (1971). *Imperialism*, London and Basingstoke: Macmillan.

Darwin, C. (1888). *The Origin of Species*, 6th edn, London: John Murray.

Darwin, C. (1948). *The Origin of Species and The Descent of Man*, New York: Modern Library.

Darwin, C. (1970). *The Origin of Species*, Harmondsworth: Penguin.

Davidson, P. (1990). *Bookmark: The Storyteller*, BBC 2 Television, 7 March 1990.

Davis, D. B. (1966). *The Problem of Slavery in Western Culture*, Ithaca: Cornell University Press.

Deleuze, G. and Guattari, F. (1983). *Anti-Oedipus: Capitalism and Schizophrenia*, Minneapolis: University of Minnesota Press.

Delgado, R. (1987). 'The Ethereal Scholar: Does Critical Legal Studies Have What Minorities Want?', *Harvard Civil Rights – Civil Liberties Law Review*, 22 (2): 301–22.

213

Derrida, J. (1982). *Margins of Philosophy*, Chicago: The University of Chicago Press.

Derrida, J. (1990). 'Force of Law: "The Mystical Foundation of Authority"', *Cardozo Law Review* 11: 919–1046.

⊣ Diamond, S. (1973). 'The Rule of Law Versus the Order of Custom', in D. Black and M. Mileski (eds), *The Social Organisation of Law*, New York and London: Seminar Press.

Dicey, A. V. (1962). *Lectures on the Relation Between Law and Public Opinion in England During the Nineteenth Century*, 2nd edn, London: Macmillan.

Dicey, A. V. (1982). *Introduction to the Study of the Law of the Constitution* (Reprint of the 8th edition of 1915), Indianapolis: Liberty Classics.

Diderot, D. (1950). *Le Neveu de Rameau*, Genève: Droz.

Dingwall, R. (1988). 'Empowerment or Enforcement? Some Questions about Power and Control in Divorce Mediation', in R. Dingwall and J. M. Eekelaar (eds), *Divorce Mediation and the Legal Process: British Practice and International Experience*, Oxford: Oxford University Press.

Donzelot, J. (1980). *The Policing of Families: Welfare versus the State*, London: Hutchinson.

Douglas, M. (1970). *Purity and Danger: An Analysis of Concepts of Pollution and Taboo*, Harmondsworth: Penguin.

Douzinas, C. and Warrington, R., with McVeigh, S. (1991). *Postmodern Jurisprudence: The Law of Text in the Texts of Law*, London: Routledge.

DuBow, F. (1987a). 'Overview of Community Boards', in F. DuBow (ed.), *Conflicts and Community: A Study of the San Francisco Community Boards*, Draft. Chicago Center for Research in Law and Justice, The University of Illinois at Chicago.

DuBow, F. (1987b). 'Uniqueness' and 'Impact', in ibid.

DuBow, F. (1987c). 'Conflict Resolution', in ibid.

DuBow, F. (1987d). 'Volunteer Development', in ibid.

Dumont, L. (1965). 'The Modern Conception of the Individual: Notes on its Genesis and that of Concomitant Institutions', *Contributions to Indian Sociology*, VIII: 13–61.

Duncanson, I. (1989). 'Power, Interpretation and Ronald Dworkin', *University of Tasmania Law Review*, 9 (3): 278–301.

Durkheim, E. (1983). *Durkheim and the Law*, Oxford: Martin Robertson.

Duxbury, N. (1987). *Phenomenological Jurisprudence: An Ontological Sketch*, Ph.D. Thesis submitted to the London School of Economics and Political Science, November 1987.

Duxbury, N. (1989). 'Exploring Legal Tradition: Psychoanalytical Theory and Roman Law in Modern Continental Jurisprudence', *Legal Studies*, 9 (1): 84–98.

Duxbury, N. (1990). 'Back to the Middle Ages: Review of Pierre Legendre, *Le Désir Politique de Dieu . . .*', *International Journal for the Semiotics of Law*, III (7): 65–79.

Dworkin, R. (1968). 'Is Law a System of Rules?', in R. J. Summers (ed.), *Essays in Legal Philosophy*, Oxford: Basil Blackwell.

Dworkin, R. (1977). *Taking Rights Seriously*, London: Duckworth.

⊣ Dworkin, R. (1986). *Law's Empire*, London: Fontana.

Eliade, M. (1963). *Myth and Reality*, New York: Harper & Row.

BIBLIOGRAPHY

Eliade, M. (1965). *The Myth of the Eternal Return or, Cosmos and History*, Princeton: Princeton University Press.

Eliade, M. (1968). *Myths, Dreams and Mysteries: The Encounter Between Contemporary Faiths and Archaic Reality*, Glasgow: Collins.

Elias, N. (1978). *The Civilizing Process; Volume 1: The History of Manners*, New York: Urizon Books.

Eliot, T. S. (1935). *Murder in the Cathedral*, London: Faber & Faber.

Ellmann, R. (1988). *Oscar Wilde*, London: Penguin.

Evans-Pritchard, E. E. (1937). *Witchcraft, Oracles and Magic among the Azande*, Oxford: Clarendon Press.

Ewald, F. (1990). 'Norms, Discipline, and the Law', *Representations*, 30 (Spring): 138–61.

Fabian, J. (1983). *Time and the Other: How Anthropology Makes its Object*, New York: Columbia University Press.

Fanon, F. (1967). *Black Skin, White Masks*, New York: Grove Press.

Faris, J. C. (1973). 'Pax Britannica and the Sudan: S. F. Nadel', in T. Asad (ed.), *Anthropology and the Colonial Encounter*, London: Ithaca Press.

Feldman, B. and Richardson, R. D. (1972). *The Rise of Modern Mythology 1680–1860*, Bloomington: Indiana University Press.

Ferguson, A. (1966). *An Essay on the History of Civil Society 1767*, Edinburgh: Edinburgh University Press.

Fish, S. (1989). *Doing What Comes Naturally: Change, Rhetoric, and the Practice of Theory in Literary and Legal Studies*, Oxford: Clarendon Press.

Fitzpatrick, P. (1983). 'Law, Plurality and Underdevelopment', in D. Sugarman (ed.), *Legality, Ideology and the State*, London and New York: Academic Press.

Fitzpatrick, P. (1984). 'Traditionalism and Traditional Law', *Journal of African Law*, 28: 20–7.

Fitzpatrick, P. (1985). 'Is it Simple to be a Marxist in Legal Anthropology?', *Modern Law Review*, 48: 472–85.

Fitzpatrick, P. (1987). 'Racism and the Innocence of Law', in P. Fitzpatrick and A. Hunt (eds), *Critical Legal Studies*, Oxford: Basil Blackwell.

Fitzpatrick, P. (1988a). 'Legalidade terminal: a situação em Inglaterra', *Vértice, II Série*, 5 (August): 39–41.

Fitzpatrick, P. (1988b). 'The Rise and Rise of Informalism', in R. Matthews (ed.), *Informal Justice?*, London: Sage.

Fitzpatrick, P. (1991). 'The Abstracts and Brief Chronicles of the Times: Supplementing Jurisprudence', in P. Fitzpatrick (ed.), *Dangerous Supplements: Resistance and Renewal in Jurisprudence*, London: Pluto Press; Durham: Duke University Press.

Fitzpatrick, P. (1992). 'The Impossibility of Popular Justice', *Social and Legal Studies* 1: 199–215.

Foucault, M. (1967). *Madness and Civilization: A History of Insanity in the Age of Reason*, London: Tavistock.

Foucault, M. (1970). *The Order of Things: An Archeology of the Human Sciences*, London: Tavistock.

Foucault, M. (1972). *The Archeology of Knowledge*, London: Tavistock.

Foucault, M. (1977). *Language, Counter-Memory, Practice: Selected Essays and Interviews*, Oxford: Basil Blackwell.

Foucault, M. (1979a). *Discipline and Punish: The Birth of the Prison*, Harmondsworth: Penguin.

Foucault, M. (1979b). 'Governmentality', *I & C*, 6 (Autumn): 5–21.

Foucault, M. (1979c). 'My Body, This Paper, This Fire', *Oxford Literary Review*, 4 (1): 9–28.

Foucault, M. (1980). *Power/Knowledge: Selected Interviews and Other Writings 1972–1977*, Brighton: Harvester Press.

Foucault, M. (1981). *The History of Sexuality, Volume I: An Introduction*, Harmondsworth: Penguin.

Foucault, M. (1982). 'Afterword: The Subject and Power', in H. L. Dreyfus and P. Rabinow (eds), *Michel Foucault: Beyond Structuralism and Hermeneutics*, Brighton: Harvester Press.

Foucault, M. (1987). *The Use of Pleasure: The History of Sexuality: Volume Two*, Harmondsworth: Penguin.

Foucault, M. (1988). 'The Political Technology of Individuals', in L. H. Martin, H. Gutman and P. H. Hutton (eds), *Technologies of the Self: A Seminar with Michel Foucault*, London: Tavistock.

Frazer, J. G. (1914). *The Golden Bough*, 3rd edn, London: Macmillan.

Freud, S. (1949). *An Outline of Psycho-Analysis*, New York: W. W. Norton.

Freud, S. (1950). *Totem and Taboo*, New York: W. W. Norton.

Freud, S. (1985). *Civilization and its Discontents* in *Volume 12: Civilization, Society and Religion . . . and Other Works*, London: Penguin.

Freud, S. (n.d.). *Moses and Monotheism*, New York: Random House, Vintage Books.

Fryer, P. (1988). *Staying Power: The History of Black People in Britain*, London: Pluto Press.

Galanter, M. (1980). 'Legality and Its Discontents: A Preliminary Assessment of Current Theories of Legalization and Delegalization', in E. Blankenburg, E. Klausa and H. Rottleuthner (eds), *Alternative Rechtsformen und Alternativen zum Recht Jahrbuch für Rechtssoziologie und Rechtstheorie, Band VI*, Opladen: Westdeutscher Verlag.

Galligan, D. J. (1982). 'Judicial Review and the Textbook Writers', *Oxford Journal of Legal Studies*, 2: 257–76.

Geertz, C. (1983). *Local Knowledge: Further Essays in Interpretive Anthropology*, New York: Basic Books.

Gellner, E. (1983). *Nations and Nationalism*, Oxford: Basil Blackwell.

Giddens, A. (1981). *A Contemporary Critique of Historical Materialism: Volume I Power, Property and the State*, London and Basingstoke: Macmillan.

Gilroy, P. (1987). *'There Ain't No Black in the Union Jack': The Cultural Politics of 'Race' and Nation*, London: Hutchinson.

Gluckman, M. (1968). 'Magic, Sorcery and Witchcraft', in G. D. Mitchell (ed.), *A Dictionary of Sociology*, London: Routledge & Kegan Paul, 110–11.

Goldberg, D. T. (in press). *Racist Culture*, New York: Blackwell Publishers.

Goodrich, P. (1987). *Legal Discourse: Studies in Linguistics, Rhetoric and Legal Analysis*, London: Macmillan.

Goodrich, P. (1990). *Languages of Law: From Logics of Memory to Nomadic Masks*, London: Weidenfeld & Nicolson.

Goodrich, P. and Hachamovitch, Y. (1991). 'Time Out of Mind: An Introduction to the Semiotics of Common Law', in P. Fitzpatrick (ed.), *Dangerous Supplements: Resistance and Renewal in Jurisprudence*, London: Pluto Press; Durham: Duke University Press.

Goody, J. (1976). *Production and Reproduction: A Comparative Study of the Domestic Domain*, Cambridge: Cambridge University Press.

Gould, S. J. (1987). *Time's Arrow Time's Cycle: Myth and Metaphor in the Discovery of Geological Time*, Cambridge: Harvard University Press.

Gramsci, A. (1957). *The Modern Prince and Other Writings*, New York: International Publishers.

Guardian, The (1989/90). Newspaper of 21 September 1989 and 22 November 1990.

Gurvitch, G. (1947). *Sociology of Law*, London: Routledge & Kegan Paul.

Habermas, J. (1971). *Toward a Rational Society: Student Protest, Science and Politics*, London: Heinemann.

Habermas, J. (1974). *Theory and Practice*, London: Heinemann.

Habermas, J. (1976). *Legitimation Crisis*, London: Heinemann.

Habermas, J. (1979). *Communication and the Evolution of Society*, London: Heinemann.

Habermas, J. (1985). 'Modernity – An Incomplete Project', in H. Foster (ed.), *Postmodern Culture*, London: Pluto Press.

Habermas, J. (1987). *The Philosophical Discourse of Modernity: Twelve Lectures*, Cambridge: Polity Press.

Habermas, J. (1990). *The New Conservatism: Cultural Criticism and the Historians' Debate*, Cambridge: Polity Press.

Hagerström, A. (1953). *Inquiry into the Nature of Law and Morals*, Stockholm: Almqvist & Wiksell.

Hale, M. (1677). *The Primitive Origination of Mankind, Considered and Examined According to the Light of Nature*, London: W. Godbid.

Haller, J. S. (1975). *Outcasts from Evolution: Scientific Attitudes of Racial Inferiority, 1859–1900*, New York: McGraw-Hill.

Hamilton, E. (1953). *Mythology*, New York: Mentor Books.

Harrington, C. B. and Merry, S. E. (1988). 'Ideological Production: The Making of Community Mediation', *Law & Society Review*, 22: 709–35.

Harrington, C. B. and Yngvesson, B. (1990). 'Interpretive Sociological Research', *Law & Social Inquiry*, 15 (1): 135–48.

Harris, J. W. (1980). *Legal Philosophies*, London: Butterworths.

Hart, H. L. A. (1954a). 'Introduction' to J. Austin, *The Province of Jurisprudence Determined and The Uses of the Study of Jurisprudence*, London: Weidenfeld & Nicolson.

Hart, H. L. A. (1954b). 'Definition and Theory in Jurisprudence', *Law Quarterly Review*, 70: 37–60.

Hart, H. L. A. (1961). *The Concept of Law*, London: Oxford University Press.

Hart, H. L. A. (1982). *Essays on Bentham: Studies in Jurisprudence and Political Theory*, Oxford: Clarendon Press.

Hart, H. L. A. (1983). *Essays in Jurisprudence and Philosophy*, Oxford: Clarendon Press.

Hart, H. L. A. (1987). 'Comment', in R. Gavison (ed.), *Issues in Con-*

temporary Legal Philosophy: The Influence of H. L. A. Hart, Oxford: Clarendon Press.

Hawkins, K. (1986). *Handbook for Conciliation Trainers*, San Francisco: Community Board Center for Policy and Training.

Hay, D. (1975). 'Property, Authority and the Criminal Law', in D. Hay *et al.* (eds), *Albion's Fatal Tree: Crime and Society in Eighteenth Century England*, London: Allen Lane.

Hayek, F. A. von (1944). *The Road to Serfdom*, London: Routledge.

Hegel, G. W. F. (1977). *Phenomenology of Spirit*, Oxford: Clarendon Press.

Henry, S. (1982). 'Factory Law: The Changing Disciplinary Technology of Industrial Social Control', *International Journal of the Sociology of Law*, 10 (4): 365–83.

Henry, S. (1983). *Private Justice: Towards Integrated Theorizing in the Sociology of Law*, London: Routledge & Kegan Paul.

Hill, C. (1955). *The English Revolution 1640*, 3rd edn, London: Lawrence & Wishart.

Hill, C. (1969). *The Pelican Economic History of Britain Volume 2: 1530–1780: Reformation to Industrial Revolution*, Harmondsworth: Penguin.

Hindess, B. and Hirst, P. (1977). *Mode of Production and Social Formation: An Auto-critique of Pre-Capitalist Modes of Production*, London: Macmillan.

Hirst, P. and Jones, P. (1987). 'The Critical Resources of Established Jurisprudence', in P. Fitzpatrick and A. Hunt (eds), *Critical Legal Studies*, Oxford: Basil Blackwell.

Hobbes, T. (1952). *Leviathan*, Chicago: Encyclopaedia Britannica.

Hobsbawm, E. J. (1990). *Nations and Nationalism Since 1780: Programme, Myth, Reality*, Cambridge: Cambridge University Press.

Hocart, A. M. (1927). *Kingship*, London: Oxford University Press.

Hodgen, M. T. (1964). *Early Anthropology in the Sixteenth and Seventeenth Centuries*, Philadelphia: University of Pennsylvania Press.

Hoebel, E. A. (1954). *The Law of Primitive Man: A Study in Comparative Legal Dynamics*, Cambridge: Harvard University Press.

Holdsworth, W. (1952). *A History of English Law*, Volume XIII, London: Methuen and Sweet & Maxwell.

Holland, T. E. (1924). *The Elements of Jurisprudence*, Clarendon Press: Oxford.

Horwitz, M. J. (1977). *The Transformation of American Law, 1780–1860*, Clarendon Press: Oxford.

⅄Hulme, P. (1990). 'The Spontaneous Hand of Nature: Savagery, Colonialism and the Enlightenment', in P. Hulme and L. Jordanova (eds), *The Enlightenment and its Shadows*, London: Routledge.

Hume, D. (1888). *A Treatise of Human Nature*, Oxford: Clarendon Press.

Hunt, A. (1990). 'Rights and Social Movements: Counter-Hegemonic Strategies', *Journal of Law and Society*, 17 (3): 309–28.

Hunt, A. and Kerruish, V. (in press). 'Dworkin's Dutiful Daughters: Gender Discrimination in Law's Empire', in A. Hunt (ed.), *Reading Dworkin Critically*, New York: Berg.

Isaacs, J. (ed.) (1980). *Australian Dreaming: 40,000 Years of Aboriginal History*, Sydney: Lansdowne Press.

Jakubowski, F. (1976). *Ideology and Superstructure in Historical Materialism*, London: Allison & Busby.

Jones, G. (1980). *Social Darwinism and English Thought: The Interaction Between Biological and Social Theory*, Brighton: Harvester.

Jordanova, L. J. (1980). 'Natural Facts: A Historical Perspective on Science and Sexuality', in C. P. MacCormack and M. Strathern (eds), *Nature, Culture and Gender*, Cambridge: Cambridge University Press.

Kafka, F. (1961). *Metamorphosis and Other Stories*, Harmondsworth: Penguin.

Kafka, F. (1988a). 'The Problem of Our Laws', in *The Collected Short Stories of Franz Kafka*, London: Penguin.

Kafka, F. (1988b). *The Trial*, in *The Collected Novels of Franz Kafka*, London: Penguin.

Kelley, D. R. (1984a). *Historians and the Law in Postrevolutionary France*, Princeton: Princeton University Press.

Kelley, D. R. (1984b). *History, Law and the Human Sciences: Medieval and Renaissance Perspectives*, London: Variorum Reprints.

Kelsen, H. (1961). *General Theory of Law and State*, New York: Russell & Russell.

Kelsen, H. (1967). *The Pure Theory of Law*, Berkeley: University of California Press.

Kelsey, J. (1990). *A Question of Honour? Labour and the Treaty 1984–1989*, Wellington: Allen & Unwin.

Kiernan, V. G. (1972). *The Lords of Human Kind*, Harmondsworth: Penguin.

Klare, K. (1979). 'Law-Making as Praxis', *Telos*, 40: 123–35.

Knox, R. (1862). *The Races of Men: A Philosophical Enquiry into the Influences of Race Over the Destinies of Nations*, 2nd edn, London: Henry Renshaw.

Konecni, V. J. and Ebbesen, E. B. (1984). 'The Mythology of Legal Decision Making', *International Journal of Law and Psychiatry*, 7: 5–18.

Kronman, A. T. (1983). *Max Weber*, London: Edward Arnold.

Kuper, A. (1988). *The Invention of Primitive Society: Transformation of an Illusion*, London: Routledge.

Landau, M. (1991). *Narratives of Human Evolution*, New Haven: Yale University Press.

Lasch, C. (1977). *Haven in a Heartless World: The Family Besieged*, New York: Basic Books.

Leach, E. (1969). *Genesis as Myth and Other Essays*, London: Jonathan Cape.

Leach, E. (1974). *Lévi-Strauss*, Glasgow: Fontana.

Lefort, C. (1986). *The Political Forms of Modern Society: Bureaucracy, Democracy, Totalitarianism*, Cambridge: Polity Press.

Legendre, P. (1974). *L'Amour du Censeur. Essai sur l'Ordre Dogmatique*, Paris: Seuil.

Legendre, P. (1976). *Jouir du Pouvoir. Traité de la Bureaucratie Patriote*, Paris Éditions du Minuit.

Legendre, P. (1990). 'The Lost Temporality of Law', *Law and Critique*, 1 (1): 3–20. Interview conducted by P. Goodrich and R. Warrington.

Leith, P. (1988). 'Common Usage, Certainty and Computing', in P. Leith and P. Ingram (eds), *The Jurisprudence of Orthodoxy: Queen's University Essays on H. L. A. Hart*, London: Routledge.

Lempert, R. and Sanders, J. (1986). *An Invitation to Law and Social Science: Desert, Disputes and Distribution*, New York: Longman.

Lenoble, J. and Ost, F. (1980). *Droit, Mythe et Raison. Essai sur la Dérive Mytho-Logique de la Rationalité Juridique*, Brussels: Facultés Universitaires Saint-Louis.

Lenoble, J. and Ost, F. (1986). 'Founding Myths in Legal Rationality', *Modern Law Review*, 49: 530–44.

Leopardi, G. (1966). *Selected Prose and Poetry*, London: Oxford University Press.

Levinas, E. (1979). *Totality and Infinity: An Essay on Exteriority*, The Hague: Martinus Nijhoff.

Lévi-Strauss, C. (1968). *Structural Anthropology*, Harmondsworth: Penguin.

√Lévi-Strauss, C. (1986). *The Raw and the Cooked: Introduction to a Science of Mythology: I*, Harmondsworth: Penguin.

√Lévi-Strauss, C. (1987). *Anthropology and Myth: Lectures 1951–1982*, Oxford: Basil Blackwell.

Lieberman, D. (1989). *The Province of Legislation Determined: Legal Theory in Eighteenth-century Britain*, Cambridge: Cambridge University Press.

Lloyd, D. and Freeman, M. D. A. (1985). *Lloyd's Introduction to Jurisprudence: Fifth Edition*, London: Stevens.

Locke, J. (1965). 'The Second Treatise of Government', in *Two Treatises of Government*, New York: New American Library.

Long, E. (1774). *The History of Jamaica*, 3 vols, London: T. Lowndes.

Lovejoy, A. O. (1966). *The Great Chain of Being: A Study in the History of an Idea*, Cambridge: Harvard University Press.

Lugard, Lord (1965). *The Dual Mandate in British Tropical Africa*, 5th edn, London: Frank Cass.

Lukes, S. and Scull, A. (1983). 'Introduction' to E. Durkheim, *Durkheim and the Law*, Oxford: Martin Robertson.

Lyotard, J. F. (1984). *The Postmodern Condition: A Report on Knowledge*, Minneapolis: University of Minnesota Press.

MacCormick, N. (1981). *H. L. A. Hart*, London: Edward Arnold.

MacCormick, N. (1987). 'Comment', in R. Gavison (ed.), *Issues in Contemporary Legal Philosophy: The Influence of H. L. A. Hart*, Oxford: Clarendon Press.

MacIntyre, A. (1981). *After Virtue: A Study in Moral Theory*, London: Duckworth.

Mackenzie, J. M. (1984). *Propaganda and Empire: The Manipulation of British Public Opinion, 1880–1960*, Manchester: Manchester University Press.

Maine, H. (1897). *Lectures on the Early History of Institutions*, 7th edn, London: Murray.

Maine, H. (1931). *Ancient Law*, London: Oxford University Press.

Malinowski, B. (1932). *The Sexual Life of Savages*, 3rd edn, London: Routledge & Kegan Paul.

Malinowski, B. (1954). *Magic, Science and Religion and Other Essays*, Garden City: Doubleday.

Malinowski, B. (1961). *Argonauts of the Western Pacific*, New York: E. P. Dutton.

Manganyi, N. C. (1985). 'Making Strange: Race, Science and Ethno-psychiatric Discourse', in F. Baker *et al.* (eds), *Europe and Its Others: Volume One*, Colchester: University of Essex.

Mann, M. (1986). *The Sources of Social Power: Volume 1: A History of Power from the Beginning to A. D. 1760*, Cambridge: Cambridge University Press.

Marshall, P. J. and Williams, G. (1982). *The Great Map of Mankind: British Perceptions of the World in the Age of Enlightenment*, London: J. M. Dent & Sons.

Marx, K. (1959). *Capital I*, Moscow: Foreign Languages Publishing House.

Marx, K. (1969). *Karl Marx on Colonialism and Modernization*, New York: Anchor Books.

Marx, K. (1973). *Grundrisse: Foundations of the Critique of Political Economy*, Harmondsworth: Penguin.

Marx, K. and Engels, F. (1957). *On Religion*, Moscow: Foreign Languages Publishing House.

Marx, K. and Engels, F. (1974). *The German Ideology Part I*, London: Lawrence & Wishart.

Matthews, R. (1988). 'Reassessing Informal Justice', in R. Matthews (ed.), *Informal Justice?*, London: Sage.

Mayhew, L. H. (1971). 'Stability and Change in Legal Systems', in B. Barber and A. Inkeles (eds), *Stability and Social Change*, Boston: Little, Brown & Company.

Meek, R. L. (1976). *Social Science and the Ignoble Savage*, Cambridge: Cambridge University Press.

Merry, S. E. (1982). 'The Social Organization of Mediation in Non-industrial Societies: Implications for Informal Community Justice in America', in R. Abel (ed.), *The Politics of Informal Justice: Volume 2: Comparative Perspectives*, New York: Academic Press.

Merry, S. E. (1990). *Getting Justice and Getting Even: Legal Consciousness Among Working-Class Americans*, Chicago: University of Chicago Press.

Merton, R. K. (1981). 'Foreword: Remarks on Theoretical Pluralism', in P. M. Blau and R. K. Merton (eds), *Continuities in Structural Inquiry*, London: Sage.

Michener, R. E. (1982). 'Foreword', in A. V. Dicey, *Introduction to the Study of the Law of the Constitution*, Indianapolis: Liberty Classics.

Mill, J. S. (1962). *On Liberty*, in *Utilitarianism, On Liberty, Essay on Bentham*, n. p. : Fontana.

Milsom, S. F. C. (1981). 'The Nature of Blackstone's Achievement', *Oxford Journal of Legal Studies*, 1 (1): 1–12.

Minson, J. (1985). *Genealogies of Morals: Nietzsche, Foucault, Donzelot and the Eccentricity of Ethics*, Basingstoke and London: Macmillan.

Moles, R. N. (1987). *Definition and Rule in Legal Theory: A Reassessment of H. L. A. Hart and the Positivist Tradition*, Oxford: Basil Blackwell.

Montaigne, M. de (1978). 'Des Cannibales', *Essais*, Paris: Presses Universitaires de France, chapitre XXXI.

221

Montesquieu, Baron De (1949). *The Spirit of the Laws*, New York: Hafner Press.

Morison, W. L. (1982). *John Austin*, London: Edward Arnold.

Morrall, J. B. (1980). *Political Thought in Medieval Times*, Toronto: University of Toronto Press.

Mosse, G. (1978). *Towards the Final Solution: A History of European Racism*, London: Dent.

Munz, P. (1973). *When the Golden Bough Breaks: Structuralism or Typology?*, London: Routledge & Kegan Paul.

Nader, L. (1988). 'The ADR Explosion – The Implications of Rhetoric in Legal Reform', *Windsor Yearbook of Access to Justice*, 8: 269–91.

√Nandy, A. (1983). *The Intimate Enemy: Loss and Recovery of Self Under Colonialism*, Delhi: Oxford University Press.

Nelken, D. (1981). 'The "Gap Problem" in the Sociology of Law: A Theoretical Review', *Windsor Yearbook of Access to Justice*, 1: 35–61.

Nelken, D. (1989). 'The Truth about Law's Truth', *U. C. L. Working Papers No. 7*, London: University College London, Faculty of Laws.

√Newman, G. (1988). *The Rise of English Nationalism: a Cultural History 1740–1830*, London: Weidenfeld & Nicolson.

Newman, K. S. (1983). *Law and Economic Organisation; A Comparative Study of Preindustrial Societies*, Cambridge: Cambridge University Press.

Nietzsche, F. (1956). *The Genealogy of Morals* in *The Birth of Tragedy and The Genealogy of Morals*, New York: Doubleday.

Nietzsche, F. (1968). *Twilight of the Idols* in *Twilight of the Idols and The Anti-Christ*, Harmondsworth: Penguin.

Nietzsche, F. (1974). *The Gay Science*, New York: Random House.

O'Donovan, K. (1985). *Sexual Divisions in Law*, London: Weidenfeld & Nicolson.

O'Farrell, C. (1989). *Foucault: Historian or Philosopher?*, Basingstoke: Macmillan.

Paley, W. (1828). *Moral and Political Philosophy* in *The Works of William Paley, D. D.*, Volume I, London: J. F. Dove.

Pashukanis, E. B. (1978). *Law and Marxism: A General Theory*, London: Ink Links.

Ӿ Pawlisch, H. S. (1985). *Sir John Davies and the Conquest of Ireland: A Study in Legal Imperialism*, Cambridge: Cambridge University Press.

Pears, D. (1971). *Wittgenstein*, London: Fontana/Collins.

Phillips, M. (1981). 'Justice that Obeys the Prison Rules', *Guardian*, 19 August 1981, 13.

Piddington, R. (1957). 'Malinowski's Theory of Needs', in R. Firth (ed.), *Man and Culture: An Evaluation of the Work of Bronislaw Malinowski*, London: Routledge & Kegan Paul.

Pocock, J. G. A. (1967). *The Ancient Constitution and the Feudal Law: A Study of English Historical Thought in the Seventeenth Century*, New York: Norton.

Poliakov, L. (1974). *The Aryan Myth: A History of Racist and Nationalist Ideas in Europe*, London: Chatto & Windus, and Heinemann, for Sussex University Press.

Pope, A. (1950). *An Essay on Man*, London: Methuen.

Pospisil, L. (1971). *Anthropology of Law: A Comparative Theory*, New York: Harper & Row.

Poulantzas, N. (1978). *State, Power, Socialism*, London: New Left Books.

Puech, H.-C. (1957). 'Gnosis and Time', in H. Corbin *et al.*, *Man and Time: Papers from the Eranos Yearbooks*, New York: Pantheon.

Rackett, T. (1985). 'Racist Social Fantasy and Paranoia', in F. Barker *et al.* (eds), *Europe and its Others: Volume Two*, Colchester: University of Essex.

Ranger, T. (1983). 'The Invention of Tradition in Colonial Africa', in E. Hobsbawm and T. Ranger (eds), *The Invention of Tradition*, Cambridge: Cambridge University Press.

Raz, J. (1980). *The Concept of a Legal System: An Introduction to the Theory of Legal System*, 2nd edn, Oxford: Clarendon Press.

Riley, P. (1986). *The General Will Before Rousseau: The Transformation of the Divine into the Civic*, Princeton: Princeton University Press.

Robinson, O. F., Fergus, T. D. and Gordon, W. M. (1985). *An Introduction to European Legal History*, Abingdon: Professional Books.

Rogers, J. D. (1987). *Crime, Justice and Society in Colonial Sri Lanka*, London: Curzon Press.

Rose, N. (1979). 'The Psychological Complex: Mental Measurement and Social Administration', *Ideology & Consciousness*, 5 (Spring): 5–68.

Rousseau, J. J. (1986). *The Social Contract and Discourses*, London: Dent.

Sahlins, M. (1976). *Culture and Practical Reason*, Chicago: University of Chicago Press.

Said, E. W. (1985). *Orientalism*, Harmondsworth: Penguin.

Sajo, A. (1990). 'New Legalism in East Central Europe: Law as an Instrument of Social Transformation', *Journal of Law and Society*, 17 (3): 329–44.

Sampford, C. (1989). *The Disorder of Law: A Critique of Legal Theory*, Oxford: Basil Blackwell.

Sarat, A. (1990). '"The Law Is All Over": Power, Resistance and the Legal Consciousness of the Welfare Poor', *Yale Journal of Law & the Humanities*, 2 (2): 343–79.

Sargent, N. C. (1991). 'Labouring in the Shadow of the Law: A Canadian Perspective on the Possibilities and Perils of Legal Studies', *Law in Context*, 9 (2): 65–86.

Sartre, J.-P. (1956). *Being and Nothingness*, New York: Philosophical Library.

Saussure, F. de (1966). *Course in General Linguistics*, New York: McGraw-Hill.

Savigny, F. C. von (1831). *Of the Vocation of Our Age for Legislation and Jurisprudence*, London: privately published.

Sedley, S. (1987). 'Judicial Review: Sounding the Retreat', *Socialist Lawyer*, 2: 10–12.

Sedley, S. (1988). 'Hidden Agendas: The Growth of Public Law in Britain and Canada', in Institute of Comparative Law Waseda University (ed.), *Law in East and West*, Tokyo: Waseda University Press.

Sheldrake, R. (1981). *A New Science of Life: The Hypothesis of Formative Causation*, London: Blond & Briggs.

223

Shewring, W. (1980). *Homer: The Odyssey*, Oxford: Oxford University Press.

Shonholtz, R. (1984). 'Neighbourhood Justice Systems: Work, Structure and Guiding Principles', *Mediation Quarterly*, 5: 3–30.

Shonholtz, R. (1987). 'The Citizens' Role in Justice: Building a Primary Justice and Prevention System at the Neighborhood Level', *Annals, AAPSS*, 494: 42–52.

Simpson, A. W. B. (1987). *Legal Theory and Legal History: Essays on the Common Law*, London: Hambledon.

Skillen, A. (1977). *Ruling Illusions: Philosophy and the Social Order*, Hassocks: Harvester.

Smith, A. (1978). *Lectures on Jurisprudence*, Oxford: Clarendon Press.

Smith, A. D. (1986). *The Ethnic Origins of Nations*, Oxford: Basil Blackwell.

Smith, J. C. (1983). 'The Sword and Shield of Perseus: Some Mythological Dimensions of the Law', *International Journal of Law and Psychiatry*, 6: 235–61.

Smith, J. C. (1984). 'Gods and Goddesses of the Quadrant: Some Further Thoughts on the Mythological Dimensions of the Law', *International Journal of Law and Psychiatry*, 7: 219–47.

Spencer, H. (1885). *Political Institutions: Being Part V of the Principles of Sociology*, London: Williams and Norgate.

Spencer, H. (1972). *On Social Evolution: Selected Writings*, Chicago: University of Chicago Press.

Spivak, G. C. (1988). 'Can the Subaltern Speak?', in C. Nelson and L. Grossberg (eds), *Marxism and the Interpretation of Culture*, Urbana: University of Illinois Press.

Stein, P. (1980). *Legal Evolution: The Story of an Idea*, Cambridge: Cambridge University Press.

Stepan, N. (1982). *The Idea of Race in Science: Great Britain 1800–1960*, London: Macmillan.

Stokes, E. (1959). *The English Utilitarians and India*, Oxford: Clarendon Press.

Stone, J. (1964). *Legal Systems and Lawyers' Reasoning*, London: Stevens.

Stone, J. (1966). *Social Dimensions of Law and Justice*, London: Stevens.

Strakosch, H. E. (1967). *State Absolutism and the Rule of Law: The Struggle for the Codification of Civil Law in Austria 1753–1811*, Sydney: Sydney University Press.

Strathern, M. (1985). 'Discovering "Social Control"', *Journal of Law and Society*, 12 (2): 111–34.

Strauss, L. and Cropsey, J. (1972). *History of Political Philosophy*, 2nd edn, Chicago: Rand McNally.

Sugarman, D. (1991). '"A Hatred of Disorder": Legal Science, Liberalism and Imperialism', in P. Fitzpatrick (ed.), *Dangerous Supplements: Resistance and Renewal in Jurisprudence*, London: Pluto Press; Durham: Duke University Press.

Sunkin, M. (1987). 'What is Happening to Applications for Judicial Review?', *Modern Law Review*, 50 (4): 432–67.

Tagore, R. (1926). *Stray Birds*, London: Macmillan.

Tawney, R. H. (1926). *Religion and the Rise of Capitalism*, London: John Murray.

Teitelbaum, L. E. and DuPaix, L. (1988). 'Alternative Dispute Resolution and Divorce: Natural Experimentation in Family Law', *Rutgers Law Review*, 40 (4): 1093–132.

Teubner, G. (1983). 'Substantive and Reflexive Elements in Modern Law', *Law & Society Review*, 17 (2): 239–85.

Teubner, G. (1987). 'Juridification: Concepts, Aspects, Limits, Solutions', in G. Teubner (ed.), *Juridification of Social Spheres: A Comparative Analysis in the Areas of Labor, Corporate, Antitrust and Social Welfare Law*, Berlin: Walter de Gruyter.

Teubner, G. (1989). 'How the Law Thinks: Toward a Constructivist Epistemology of Law', *Law & Society Review*, 23 (5): 728–57.

Thomas, K. (1984). *Man and the Natural World: Changing Attitudes in England 1500–1800*, Harmondsworth: Penguin.

Thompson, E. P. (1978). *The Poverty of Theory and Other Essays*, London: Merlin Press.

Thompson, J. B. (1986). 'Introduction' to C. Lefort, *The Political Forms of Modern Society: Bureaucracy, Democracy, Totalitarianism*, Cambridge: Polity Press.

Thornton, A. P. (1965). *Doctrines of Imperialism*, New York: John Wiley & Sons.

Tigar, M. E. and Levy, M. R. (1977). *Law and the Rise of Capitalism*, New York: Monthly Review Press.

Tocqueville, A. de (1862). *Democracy in America Volume II*, London: Longman, Green, Longman and Roberts.

Trigger, B. G. (1985). *Natives and Newcomers: Canada's 'Heroic Age' Reconsidered*, Kingston and Montreal: McGill–Queen's University Press.

Tuck, R. (1989). *Hobbes*, Oxford: Oxford University Press.

Tuke, S. (1964). *Description of the Retreat, an Institution near York for Insane Persons of the Society of Friends*, London: Dawsons of Pall Mall.

Turk, A. T. (1980). 'Conceptions of the Demise of Law', in P. J. Brantingham and J. M. Kreiss (eds), *Structure, Law and Power*, London: Sage.

Turner, B. (1987). 'A Note on Nostalgia', *Theory, Culture and Society*, 4, 147–56.

Ullmann, W. (1975). *Law and Politics in the Middle Ages: An Introduction to the Sources of Medieval Political Ideas*, Ithaca: Cornell University Press.

Unger, R. M. (1976). *Law in Modern Society: Toward a Criticism of Social Theory*, New York: The Free Press.

Urry, J. (1981). *The Anatomy of Capitalist Societies: The Economy, Civil Society and the State*, London: Macmillan.

Vattel, E. de (1971). 'Emer de Vattel on the Occupation of Territory', in P. D. Curtin, *Imperialism*, London: Macmillan.

Wade, E. C. S. and Bradley, A. W. (1985). *Constitutional and Administrative Law*, 10th edn, London and New York: Longman.

Walton, C. (1972). *De la Recherche du Bien: A Study of Malebranche's Science of Ethics*, The Hague: Martinus Nijhoff.

Watson, M. (1980). 'Trial by Prison Board', *New Society*, 4 December 1980, 463–4.

Weber, M. (1954). *Max Weber on Law in Economy and Society*, New York: Simon & Schuster.

Weber, M. (1968). *Economy and Society*, New York: Bedminster Press.

Westlake, J. (1971). 'John Westlake on the Title to Sovereignty', in P. D. Curtin, *Imperialism*, London and Basingstoke: Macmillan.

White, H. (1973). *Metahistory: The Historical Imagination in Nineteenth-Century Europe*, Baltimore.

White, H. (1978). *Tropics of Discourse: Essays in Cultural Criticism*, Baltimore: Johns Hopkins.

White, L. A. (1959). *The Evolution of Culture: The Development of Civilization to the Fall of Rome*, New York: McGraw-Hill.

Willey, B. (1940). *The Eighteenth Century Background: Studies on the Idea of Nature in the Thought of the Period*, London: Chatto & Windus.

Williams, R. (1983). *Keywords: A Vocabulary of Culture and Society*, London: Fontana.

Winch, P. (1958). *The Idea of a Social Science and its Relation to Philosophy*, London: Routledge & Kegan Paul.

Winn, P. A. (1991). 'Legal Ritual', *Law and Critique*, II (2): 207–32.

Wittgenstein, L. (1958). *The Blue Book* in *The Blue and Brown Books*, Oxford: Basil Blackwell.

Wittgenstein, L. (1967). *Remarks on the Foundations of Mathematics*, Oxford: Basil Blackwell.

Wittgenstein, L. (1968). *Philosophical Investigations*, Oxford: Basil Blackwell.

Wittgenstein, L. (1980). *Culture and Value*, Oxford: Basil Blackwell.

Wolf, E. R. (1982). *Europe and the People Without History*, Berkeley: University of California Press.

Worger, W. (1983). 'Workers as Criminals: The Rule of Law in Early Kimberley, 1870–1885', in F. Cooper (ed.), *Struggle for the City: Migrant Labor, Capital and the State in Urban Africa*, Beverly Hills: Sage.

Zilboorg, G. and Henry, G. (1941). *A History of Medical Psychology*, New York: Norton.

NAME INDEX

SUBJECT INDEX

alterity 180 [*see also* **other(nes)s**]
America(ns) 69–73, 75–9, 178, 202–3
anthropology 7, 101, 110, 178, 194
authority x, 11, 84, 106, 125, 148, 160–2, 201, 204, 206, 210 [*see also* **law** and administration and **sovereign(ty)**]
  and language 22, 33
  and law [*see* **law** and authority]
autopoiesis 9

cases
  Becker v Home Office and another 157
  Bromley L.B.C. v G.L.C. 156
  Chandler v Director of Public Prosecutions 156
  Payne v Lord Harris of Greenwich and another 158
  R. v Board of Visitors of H.M. Prison, The Maze, ex parte *Hone* 158–9
  R. v The Earl of Crewe ex parte *Sekgome* 109
  R. v Hull Prison Board of Visitors, ex parte *St. Germain* 157–8
  R. v Secretary of State for Foreign and Commonwealth Affairs, ex parte *Council of Civil Service Unions* 155–6
  Southern Pacific Co. v Jensen 61
centrality 16, 145, 167, 180

symbolism around 46–7, 203–4
chaos 28, 46–7, 62–5, 76, 86, 93, 108 [*see also* **nature**, state of and **savagery**]
  and myth [*see* **myth** and chaos]
Christianity 9, 18–19, 45–6, 57–8, 127–8 [*see also* **Genesis**]
civilization 50, 66, 71, 72–3, 76–7, 86–7, 94, 107–8, 117, 127–8, 131–3, 195, 203
colonialism/colonization 65–6, 80–2, 107–11, 113, 117, 135, 178, 201–3 [*see also* **America(ns)** and **imperialism**]
  and law [*see* **law** and colonialism]
Common Law 60–1, 114–15, 209
community
  and law [*see* **law** and community]
  and myth [*see* **myth** and community]
Community Boards 171–7, 179
criminal law 8, 129
custom(ary law) 60–1, 137–8, 145, 170, 193, 195

discipline 120–5, 127–31, 135–6, 148, 150–3, 157–60, 162–3, 176–9 [*see also* **law** and administration]
dispute 7, 169–80

230